Time Crunch Fitness

Quick Workouts for Busy Professionals

Mark Pasay

Visit the Official Website at: http://www.riptoned.com

Printed in the United States of America

First Printing: June 2024

Mark Pasay Publishing

Paperback ISBN: 978-1-7382660-0-5

Audiobook ISBN: 978-1-7382660-1-2

This book may be purchased for educational, business or sales promotional use. Special discounts are available on quantity purchases. For more information, please call or write.

Telephone: 1-888-552-0225 **Email:** support@riptoned.com

DISCLAIMER

While the author and publisher have strived to be as accurate and complete as possible in the creation of this book, readers are cautioned to rely on their own judgment about their individual circumstances to act accordingly.

The author and publisher are providing this information on an educational basis and will not be liable for damages arising out of, or in connection with, the use of the content in this book. This is a comprehensive limitation of liability that applies to all damages of any kind, including (without limitation) compensatory; direct, indirect or direct, indirect or consequential damages; loss of data, income or profit; loss of or damage to property and claims of third parties.

While all attempts have been made to verify the information provided in this publication, the author and publisher assume no responsibility for errors, omissions, or contrary interpretations of the subject matter herein. Any perceived slights of specific persons, peoples, or organizations are unintentional. This book details the author's own personal experiences and opinions.

You understand this book is not intended as a substitute for consultation with a licensed professional. In the event you use any of the information in this book for yourself, which is your constitutional right, the author and publisher assume no responsibility for your actions or outcomes.

Table of Contents

Time Crunch Fitness

Bonus Content

As an added bonus I have put together a special webpage filled with bonus content and materials to help you in your fitness journey:

Demonstration quick-workout exercise videos

Workout program videos

PDF guides for various fitness topics

Advanced exercises for when you're ready for the next level

Advanced exercise programs for when you need an extra challenge

More exercises and programs are being added regularly

Visit https://lift.riptoned.com/crunch or scan the QR code below for free access.

Introduction

Our lives are filled to the brim with obligations—between work, family, and run-of-the-mill maintenance, it can sometimes feel like there's no space for anything else. Despite our best attempts, our to-do lists remain stubbornly persistent in reminding us of all the things we haven't done.

I found myself in this boat recently. Upon looking at the clock one day, I realized I had spent the entire day building my online business and working with clients. The professional bullet points on my to-do list were all taken care of, but I still had several obligations to fulfill. While I was carried away at my desk, I had completely forgotten to make dinner for my two young sons. Scrambling to prepare something edible, I turned my attention to the second looming bullet point on my to-do list: working out. On this particular day, I refused to let my to-do list get the best of me. It was time to get creative.

Throwing some frozen ground beef in the microwave to thaw, I dropped to the floor and did a set of push-ups. Putting a pot of water on the stove, I did as many bodyweight jump squats as I could before the microwave timer rang out. In a frying pan, I browned the meat with tomatoes and spices before dropping to the ground for another set of push-ups. I did as many lunges as I could in my kitchen while I waited for the spaghetti sauce to simmer. Cutting up veggies and tossing a salad, I set the table before doing another set of push-ups, this time placing my hands closer together on the ground for a more intense burn in my triceps. Throwing some spaghetti into the boiling water, I did a wall sit and waited—by the time the pasta was ready, my legs were feeling the burn. With a final grate of parmesan, I called out to my boys: "Dinner time!"

It wasn't the ideal workout. Yet, I managed to get my heart beating and my body moving. When I crossed "workout" and "make dinner" off my to-do list, I felt a twinge of pride in my achievements.

Though I'm now in my late '50s, I've been on my personal fitness journey since my teenage years. I've done many forms of training over the years; gym memberships, home gym workouts, bodyweight programs, yoga, circuit training, running, hiking, biking, and just about everything else you can think of. I've been through chaotic times and calm times, times as a bachelor and times as a husband, times of sickness and times of health. From a corrective scoliosis surgery in my teens to an ACL reconstruction in my '20s to a broken neck in my '40s, one fact has always remained clear: Fitness is crucial to my quality of life.

All of my major injuries required me to start my fitness journey over from scratch. I would be lying if I told you I was always dialed in that I never missed a workout. Far from it! But, I always tried to make my fitness and health a priority, and it ultimately helped me overcome some of the lowest lows in my life. My journey was by no means a direct path—it zigged and zagged, sometimes drastically. Looking back, the most important aspects of my fitness journey weren't the lengths of my workouts or the size of my biceps. Instead, I found that traits like tenacity, resilience, and determination were some of the best muscles I had. Ultimately, my commitment to my fitness, health, and body got me through all the tough times.

You have your own journey, challenges, obstacles, goals, and dreams. Sometimes, you'll find that the going can get rough, especially in the face of a packed schedule. But, if you make the same undying commitment to yourself that I did, you can—and will—achieve your fitness goals. In the following chapters, we'll explore the various components that play a role in the dynamic between your professional life and your fitness life, including elements like:

- scheduling workouts

- creating exercise plans for all levels

- working on your fitness while in transit

- nutrition for busy professionals

Our mission over the next 10 chapters can be summed up in 1 statement: We need to redefine the meaning we ascribe to fitness. You don't need any fancy equipment or previous knowledge. All you need to start your fitness journey is a willingness to learn, an enthusiasm for your own health, and an open mind.

Chapter 1:

Maximizing Fitness in Minimal Time

With so many things to pay attention to in life, it's sometimes difficult to know what to look at. Between things like work, family obligations, and hobbies pulling you in a seemingly infinite number of directions, the prospect of fitting yet *another* activity into your schedule can feel especially daunting. This is particularly true for those who work full-time, high-stress jobs. *Self*'s fitness writer Audrey Bruno articulates these struggles succinctly (2016):

> Finding time to work out when you're really super busy can sometimes feel impossible. If you spend half your day at work, eight hours—ideally—sleeping, and a couple hours commuting, you'll probably end up using any remaining free time you have to actually, you know, unwind. Because as much as you'd like to be hitting the gym after you leave the office, it can be hard to convince yourself that it's worth it when you're totally exhausted.

After all, there are only so many hours in the day, right?

We've all been there. Some days, even the simple action of coming home from work can feel exhausting. And yet, the fact remains: Your health can't be put on hold. Nature waits for no one, and your body is no exception. These two truths—the necessity of keeping yourself healthy and the time constraint your busy schedule poses—can be tough to reconcile.

The solution to this dilemma isn't necessarily *easy*, but *it is* strikingly simple. There's only one perspective you need to reach your fitness goals, and it can be summed up in three words: Time is everything!

Understanding the Value of Time in Fitness

You've probably heard the old adage, *Time is money*. This phrase actually comes from a 1748 essay written by Benjamin Franklin called *Advice to a Young Tradesman*, in which Franklin describes the necessity of good time management. For busy businesspeople with already hectic schedules, this advice is likely already a given.

However, the value of time is even more crucial in the realm of health and fitness. All too often, our culture sees fitness and working out as something fervent, difficult, and, above all, time-consuming. In reality, this is far from the truth of the matter. In fact, some argue that a good fitness routine is actually the exact opposite: moderate, simple, and time-efficient. Coincidentally, these attributes are also exactly what's needed for sustainable, long-term habit formation.

In other words, short and sweet may be the best route for your professional, physical, and long-term health goals.

The Myth of Time-Intensive Workouts

"But won't shorter workouts affect the results I see?" I hear you ask.

This is a valid concern and one that many busy professionals struggle with when considering potential fitness alternatives. However, let's consider the bigger picture for a minute: Is working out for a short time better than not working out at all?

Though we may feel like it at times, fitness isn't a zero-sum game. An all-or-nothing mentality ultimately creates a toxic mental environment in which one small setback means the total collapse of your fitness goals and routines. Additionally, we sometimes conflate long, high-intensity workouts with better, faster health outcomes when this really isn't the case. If you're still skeptical, take it from the professionals. In an interview with Business Insider, professional trainer Chris Leach notes the misconceptions accompanying starting a new workout routine (2023):

> The phrase weight quickly lost is usually quickly regained holds a lot of truth. You might see rapid results right off the bat, but after a few weeks or months, you'll almost always become rundown, tired, and ravenously hungry. That will likely result in stopping your program and losing the results, as well.

Sometimes, adopting a fast-and-furious new workout routine can also increase your risk of overtraining. Yes, you read that right! Despite the fact that we're usually more worried about being too sedentary, overtraining poses a potential danger, especially for businesspeople or entrepreneurs who are used to powering through tough issues.

When you hear the term *overtraining*, you might think of a simple case of fatigue. While fatigue can certainly be a symptom, overtraining is actually more serious. When you take on too much physical activity too quickly, your body enters a state called catabolism. In simple terms, your body's metabolism can be separated into two parts, anabolism and catabolism, the latter of which is responsible for breaking down your body's overall mass. At first, this might sound great—if catabolism burns fat, then overtraining sounds like a good choice, right? The problem is this: During catabolism, your body also destroys muscle mass in addition to fat. If your goal is to gain muscle or get stronger, overtraining can be particularly dangerous.

Aside from the simple physiological process of catabolism, overtraining also comes with a whole host of nasty side effects (Goolsby, 2021), such as:

- performance plateaus or declines

- longer recovery times

- poor sleep quality

- lack of energy, prolonged fatigue, and lower motivation

- increase in negative feelings like anger, confusion, or depression

- increased likelihood of illness

- increased blood pressure and resting heart rate

- digestive issues

Overtraining can also increase your cortisol levels, which can augment your stress in turn. Aside from eating well, sleeping well, and allowing for sufficient recovery time, there's one huge thing you can do to fight overtraining: Cap the duration of your workout to 45 minutes, *maximum*. It might sound counterintuitive, but in this instance, working out in shorter bursts can actually boost your health outcomes more than long workouts.

Time as a Resource in Fitness

Alright, so we've established that 45 minutes per day is the most you should work out, at least at first. For busy professionals, however, even carving out 45 minutes can sometimes feel like a big ask. Luckily, there are a couple more professionally-recommended guidelines that can help you pin down the basic outline of your workout routine.

To start, the American Heart Association recommends about 150 minutes of exercise per week, or about 20 minutes every day (*American Heart Association*, 2018). Already, 20 minutes of aerobic exercise per day is far less of a daunting task. A total of 20–45 minutes per day is the guideline you should strive for when you start building your fitness routine.

Next, it's crucial to remember you don't have to knock everything out at once—shorter ten-minute bursts at multiple points throughout the day are just as effective as one half-hour session. Here, let's examine the concept of *time confetti*, a phrase coined by author Brigid Schulte; *time confetti* essentially describes "all of the tiny chunks of time you spend doing unproductive or unintentional things." Once you start looking at the breakdown of your day, you'll start to find these little pieces of time confetti everywhere. Five minutes scrolling on Instagram here, ten minutes waiting for the bus there, and suddenly you're faced with entire hours and half-hours spent doing things you don't even consciously think about! Personally, I like to do bodyweight squats and calf raises while I'm brushing my teeth. It's here, in these fleeting chunks of time confetti, when you have the opportunity to do something intentional that contributes to your fitness goals. Waiting for the coffee to brew? Try doing a couple of lunges while you wait. Mindlessly scrolling through Instagram? Take note, then put down your phone in favor of something a little more active.

It's worth saying that you'll never be able to catch every single piece of time confetti that floats your way. But, a little awareness can go a long way in minimizing time drains and maximizing intentional fitness.

Psychological Benefits of Short Workouts

Let's take a step back for a moment and consider two situations.

You wake up early in the morning, eat a quick breakfast, and head into your workday. It's a massive day, and your to-do list looks 100 miles long. After hours of problem-solving and troubleshooting, you finally head home to relax and unwind. Just as you're sitting down, you realize there's still one last thing on your to-do list: You still need to work out for at least 30 minutes. You can feel your stress levels rising, and you feel a little disappointed in yourself for having forgotten your fitness goals. After trying to silently motivate yourself for a few seconds, you finally give up and decide that you'll just make up for it with a longer workout tomorrow.

Now, think about the alternative. You wake up early in the morning and eat a quick breakfast. As you're heading into your workday, you decide to bike, even though it might take a few minutes longer. Periodically throughout your workday, you get up from your desk and do a couple of lunges and burpees to get your heart rate up, just a few minutes each time. Instead of immediately taking lunch at your workspace like you usually would, you head to the nearest flight of stairs, set your phone timer for 5 minutes, and run a couple of laps. After finally going home and sitting down, you feel satisfied about what you were able to accomplish. In addition to your work and to-do items, you were also able to get in a total of 30 minutes of exercise throughout the day. You're able to relax completely, and you go to bed feeling fulfilled, content, and present in the moment.

You probably already know what the first scenario feels like. At one point or another, we've all felt that sinking feeling in our gut when we realize how unmanageable a 30-minute workout is at the very end of an exhausting day. For long-term fitness, you can't push your workouts to the end of your to-do list; it's just too mentally taxing.

According to psychologist Dr. David Cohen, this aspect of pragmaticism is often overlooked when forming new routines or checking off items on your to-do list. When we write down big projects or tasks—like a 40-minute workout session for someone just starting their fitness journey—we often end up avoiding them because they're too overwhelming (Chunn, 2017). Instead, it's much more psychologically manageable to break those big tasks up into smaller, more detailed ones and sprinkle them throughout our day.

If you've ever played a role-playing video game, you're probably familiar with the idea of side quests: the small mini-games or tasks you do to build skill, take a break from the pressure of the main story, or just try something new. For many video game enthusiasts, the side quests are often more fun and quirky than the main story. Short workout bursts are like side quests that you do in real life, and they can even start to feel fun after a while. Doesn't that sound better than a looming, unmanageable item weighing down your to-do list?

Strategies for Effective, Short-Duration Workouts

For some, sprinting up and down a flight of stairs during a lunch break is enough. For others, however, the prospect of spontaneity throughout the day can actually be another source of stress. If this sounds like you, don't worry; there are still plenty of ways to use short workout bursts to your advantage while still maintaining a more structured schedule. Here, we'll go over the most popular structured routines for time-efficient workouts.

High-Intensity Interval Training (HIIT) Basics

In essence, *high-intensity interval training*—typically called HIIT—is "a workout method that uses repeated cycles of high and low-intensity workouts for a short period of time." The term *intensity* usually refers to your heart rate while exercising; high-intensity activities are performed closer to your maximum heart rate, while low-intensity activities are performed at a much lower heart rate. Fair warning: The foundations of HIIT require a little bit of high school algebra.

According to the American College of Sports Medicine, low-intensity activities are performed at 40–50% of your maximum heart rate, and they usually include things like walking briskly, cycling, or low-impact exercises like squats. High-intensity activities are performed at 80–90% of your maximum heart rate, and they usually include things like burpees, running, or fast rowing (Kravitz, 2014). For some reference, your maximum heart rate is calculated by subtracting your age from 220. A 50-year-old's maximum heart rate, for instance, is 170 beats per minute—or bpm—while a 30-year-old's maximum heart rate is 190 bpm (*Target Heart Rate and Estimated Maximum Heart Rate*, 2020). By extension, a low-intensity exercise would be performed at around 90 bpm, and a high-intensity exercise would be performed at around 160 bpm.

That being said, you don't always need to bust out the calculator in the middle of an exercise. Chances are, you probably already know what high- and low-intensity activities feel like. The great thing about HIIT is that the possible combinations of activities are virtually endless—if you prefer burpees to sprints, for instance, you can still use burpees as your high-intensity activity during a workout. In the coming chapters, we'll explore some potential HIIT routines to get you started.

Circuit Training for Busy Schedules

Another option for those with tight time frames is circuit training. Unlike HIIT, circuit training revolves around working out as many parts of your body in as little time as possible. This is a great option for those looking for more comprehensive, full-body workouts, and you can train both individually and in class settings.

While it can be lengthened somewhat, most circuit training routines max out at 30 minutes, and they typically either focus on time-based exercises or the number of repetitions (reps) completed. Time-based circuits will usually have you doing exercises for 30 seconds to 1 minute each, whereas rep-based circuits require a certain number of reps before moving on to the next exercise. Unlike HIIT, circuit training omits recovery time completely, meaning that you'll stay at your maximum heart rate for the duration of the circuit. This makes circuits a good option for those who want to knock out their workout all at once—as long as you don't mind a higher level of sustained intensity.

Incorporating Strength and Cardio Effectively

When you're thinking about creating a new workout routine, it's important to have all of your bases covered. This means that, while you might not be looking to have biceps like Arnold Schwarzenegger or run like Usain Bolt, it's still important to make your workouts well-rounded. In the fitness world, this is usually done by assigning different muscle groups to different days of the week, resulting in terms like *leg day*.

You might already see a problem with this system: If you don't like working out a particular area of your body, you might be inclined to start skipping workouts altogether. Shorter workout routines—particularly circuit training—avoid this pitfall by incorporating elements of strength and cardio exercises into every workout routine. While programs like HIIT can get your heart rate up and work your muscles, circuit training often intentionally incorporates strength training into your daily circuit. This ultimately means that, despite only doing a few minutes or a few reps at a time, you're working out the same muscle groups every day. Over time, this will result in better muscle growth overall.

Traditional exercises like burpees are great, but they're not the only option. Exercising outdoors or opting for more unorthodox workouts is another way to make your fitness tolerable—and sometimes even fun. Outdoor activities like hiking, swimming, or team sports like volleyball can all be adjusted to include elements of both cardio and strength training. Even better, activities like team sports or martial arts often involve other people, which can present a great way to keep yourself accountable while still having fun. Alternatively, you don't necessarily have to stick to traditional workouts— dancing, rigorous gardening, and even home remodeling can all work in your favor.

Practical Tips for Integrating Workouts Into a Hectic Lifestyle

No matter how busy you are, there will always be moments of time confetti. As long as you can grab them, you'll be able to integrate fitness into everything you do. Here, we'll talk about some of the little pieces of time confetti you can use to your advantage.

Sneaking Fitness Into Daily Activities

If you're a parent of a picky eater, you probably know the age-old trick of hiding fruits and veggies in your kid's dinner. While you might not be as resistant to working out, a slightly more sneaky conceptualization of fitness can maximize your fitness results. While you might be at a desk all day, there are still a couple of ways to do this, namely:

- Taking the stairs. Even in instances when stairs take longer than the elevator, it's still a good idea to get some extra steps in. You don't always have to run the stairs, either. While sprinting up a couple of flights can give you an extra prework boost of energy, you can also climb more slowly on days when you're feeling tired.

- Walking meetings. This is a particularly good option for people who work in office settings. For your next meeting, suggest a walk-and-talk meeting to your colleagues or employees. In addition to getting some extra steps in, you'll prompt a good fitness culture in your workplace.

- Parking farther away from your destinations. While the extra dozen or so steps you take across the parking lot may seem negligible in the grand scheme of things, parking farther away is still a good way to remind yourself of your fitness goals. Over time, these steps can add up to several more miles than you would've walked otherwise.

- Using a stability ball. It may seem like a small step, but stability balls are popular for a reason. As replacements for office chairs, stability balls can help activate your core while you work, giving you a chance to multitask during the workday.

Tailoring Workouts to Individual Needs and Preferences

Even if you're not new to structured workouts, designing and planning workouts for your own purposes can be overwhelming. Many resources online are quick to tell you exactly what to do and how to do it, but there's really no replacement for creating your own workout routine from scratch. No online blog or article can tell you exactly what you need for the most optimized workout—only you can do that. Here, we'll quickly go over the basics of creating a personalized workout routine that keeps your unique fitness goals in focus.

Customizing Workouts for Personal Goals

One of the most important parts of creating a personalized fitness routine is determining your goals. We'll discuss goals in-depth in Chapter 6, but for now, let's focus on a general overview of what your fitness goals might look like. Whether you're looking to shed some extra winter weight, gain muscle, or just take care of your body, you'll find that even your most basic goals can help narrow down the focus of your workouts. That being said, you don't have to have everything figured out from the get-go, and general fitness is a great place to start as well.

To kickstart your thought process, consider what kinds of activities you enjoy most. Do you like running or lifting weights? Maybe you're more of a laid-back yoga person, slowly building up to more difficult exercises over time. At this stage of the process, your preferences will mostly dictate the overall theme of your workouts. Doing something you genuinely enjoy, whether team sports or traditional exercises, is key to long-term, sustainable fitness routines.

From here, you can start thinking about what activities you'd like to incorporate most based on what your general goals are *and* what you like to do. The convergence of these two areas is the sweet spot when it comes to workouts, like the overlapping area in a Venn diagram. For instance, someone who enjoys playing volleyball and wants to build upper body muscle may consider something like rock climbing or weightlifting. To get the ball rolling, start by making two lists, one about things you like to do and one about your goals, and then find areas of potential overlap between the two.

Variety and Enjoyment in Workouts

When you're starting to think about creating your personalized workout routine, it's crucial to evaluate your definition of *fitness*. Workouts often evoke images of perfectly sculpted, sweat-covered people in gyms, performing vigorous high-intensity exercises without stopping. This, of course, is not how most people operate. To create something long-lasting, it's important to consider what you enjoy. Additionally, variety can be a strength in fitness, especially if you find yourself getting bored or tired of going to the gym every day. Group classes, dance, group sports, and getting outdoors can help mix up the basic stereotypical gym setting, effectively combatting boredom and promoting a sustainable routine.

Contrary to what we might think at first glance, fitness is much more than just losing weight or hitting the gym. Our misconceptions of terms like *healthy* and *fitness* can affect our attitudes toward our own health, inevitably affecting our health outcomes and general well-being. To get the most out of exercising, we first have to deconstruct our thinking about ourselves, our bodies, and our fitness goals.

This process is difficult enough on its own, but it's perhaps even more difficult for busy professionals. In the next chapter, we'll go over some methods to get you from the office to the gym.

Chapter 2

Desk to Dumbbells—Transitioning From Office to Workout Efficiently

If you're active in the business world, you've probably heard of the stereotypical personality type tropes that periodically make the rounds in human resources departments. Type A personalities are generally viewed as dominant, motivated, competitive, and achievement-oriented. Type B personalities, in contrast, are generally seen as laid-back, easy-going, and typically stress-free. As for whether this particular brand of personality typing is helpful, I can't say. But, there are certainly many professionals and business people who show typical type A traits, particularly when it comes to having an all-or-nothing mentality.

Take Nikki Bettinelli, a social media consultant and founder of social media agency NB Media. When she started her fitness journey, she threw herself into the world of health-related practices. In an interview with the Huffington Post, she stated (2020):

> I am an extremist when it comes to fitness. If I don't go full force, I don't see the point. I like to see how far I can push my body. I've done fitness model programs. A few years ago, I entered a charity boxing tournament and trained for 12 weeks, and right now, I am focused on building muscle.

Even then, after going all-in for her fitness transformation, she couldn't accomplish everything on her fitness to-do list, saying, "I definitely wish I had more time and energy for working out. I'd also like more time to add in other forms of fitness" (Khoo, 2020).

Whether you're more of a type A person or a type B, you'll ultimately never be able to dedicate all of your time or energy to your fitness journey. While going all-in isn't a particularly good or bad thing, this all-or-nothing attitude isn't the point of fitness; rather, making the decision to hit the gym in the first place should be regarded as a win. To this end, let's go over some of the ways you can make the office-to-workout transition easier on yourself.

Understanding the Office-To-Workout Transition

If you've ever tried to work out after a full day at the office, you probably already know how difficult it is. Aside from being tired, several psychological barriers can prevent you from exercising effectively. After all, being mentally present in your workout is challenging when your head is still grappling with work-related issues. Before you try to solve this problem, start by figuring out why exactly this transition is so difficult for you.

Challenges of Switching From Work to Exercise

There are several reasons why the work-to-workout transition is challenging.

Aside from personal struggles, here are a couple of common reasons why working out immediately after you've been in the office is tricky:

1. **Mental and physical tiredness:** After a long day of work, you might find yourself mentally or physically fatigued. Depending on your line of work, you may have just spent the day figuring out complex problems or dealing with tough issues, so the mental exertion of figuring out a workout routine becomes simply too much.

2. **Unpredictable, rigorous, or varying work schedules:** Full-time workdays are usually packed—full of tasks—leaving you with limited time for personal activities like working out. Finding the motivation to work out can be hard on its own, but doing so within a tight timeframe can be even harder. This issue is even more challenging to overcome if your job has fluctuating schedules from day to day, subsequently leaving you with inconsistent or incomplete workouts.

3. **Commute issues:** It may seem like a small issue on the surface, but your commute can actually play a big role in the work-to-workout transition. Dealing with rush-hour traffic or lengthy commutes can be discouraging, even more so when you've had difficult or stressful days.

4. **Home responsibilities:** In a perfect world, everything would always go to plan—You'd premake dinner before you started work in the morning, you'd never have to sweep the floor, and you'd only need to do minimal housework. In reality, this is almost never the case. Home commitments like making food, doing chores, or taking care of household administrative work are big

competitors when it comes to your attention span. In turn, fitness can take a backseat.

5. **Social and familial obligations:** After the workday or workweek, social and familial engagements often take precedence over working out, leaving you with little time for fitness. Dinner plans, family time, and other social events are usually unpredictable, which means it's sometimes difficult to stick to a strict workout routine every day.

The Role of the Work Environment in Fitness

Transitional challenges are tricky enough to navigate, but your workplace itself also plays a pivotal role in shaping your fitness. Assuming you're working at a desk for most of your workday means you're sitting in the same spot for about eight hours per day. Moreover, many of us are encouraged to do this, whether by the constant demands of productivity or by our obligations to coworkers.

On the flip side, a fitness-positive workplace culture fosters an environment conducive to physical activity. Access to amenities like on-site gyms or fitness classes can significantly impact the ease with which you engage in exercise. Flexible work schedules, support for mental well-being, and educational resources can further contribute to a holistic approach to your overall fitness. Ultimately, a workplace that actively encourages and supports physical fitness not only benefits the health of individual employees but also creates a positive organizational culture that enhances productivity.

Efficient Transition Strategies

Knowing how your workplace impacts your mental and physical accessibility to fitness, you may be wondering, "How can I make this transition easier?" There are several ways you can achieve this, but for now, we'll distinguish three categories. Pre-workout routines, technology, and mental preparation techniques can all help get you out of the office and into the right mindset for working out.

Quick Pre-Workout Routines

As it turns out, what you do before and after a workout is nearly as important as the workout itself. Think of pre-workout routines as an opportunity to give your mind and body a pep talk, hyping yourself up before you step up to the metaphorical plate. A great pre-workout routine isn't just about stretching, either. While that's certainly a part of warming up, there are several other things to think about before jumping into the heart of your workout. A good post-work, pre-workout routine might look something like this:

1. Eating a light snack, which will give you the energy and nutrients to do your best work

2. Changing into the appropriate clothes, including proper footwear like tennis shoes

3. Getting your playlist in order with whatever gets your blood pumping

4. Outlining your routine in detail, from start to finish

5. Minimizing distractions by putting your phone on *Do Not Disturb* and blocking your calendar ahead of time

Aside from getting you into the right mood, these steps will also maximize the impact of your workout and allow you to do the best job you can. Meanwhile, post-workout routines will bring you back down to earth, so to speak, enhancing your recovery and minimizing fatigue and soreness. To make the most out of your post-workout period, there are a couple of key things you can do:

- Drink water.

- Eat something small—and protein-packed.

- Stretch well.

Technology and Tools

In today's day and age, we can't seem to go anywhere without our phones. When we're working out, this can sometimes present a distraction waiting to happen. One Gmail notification, and you're completely detached from your workout. In addition to minimizing your performance, these kinds of distractions can also sometimes be a safety hazard, especially if you're trying out an exercise you've never done before.

Inversely, your phone—and other devices like smartwatches—can also be a great way to get yourself in the right headspace. In fact, you can actually use technology to your advantage by finding technological tools that motivate you and get you excited to exercise.

There are several options on this front, including—but not limited to:

- fitness apps, like Strava

- nice equipment, like smartwatches

- new and motivating tech to accessorize with like Bluetooth headphones

Psychological Preparation Techniques

Perhaps the biggest barrier you'll encounter on the road from work to workout is the mental exertion of getting yourself up and moving. Most of the time, we ascribe the term *motivation* to these kinds of problems, saying we don't feel motivated enough to exercise. Even knowing fitness is good for you, your heart may not be in it after a stressful day. While this is normal and nothing to be ashamed of, it's still important to try your best to exercise—even when you fail.

Despite the fact that the office-to-gym transition is difficult, there are several ways you can minimize the lack of motivation you feel after a long workday. For instance, you might

- schedule it on your calendar, and stick to it consistently.

- try to be consistent with your routines every day, turning your lack of motivation into an exception rather than a rule.

- keep yourself accountable by telling people about your plans or writing them down.

- dress for success by bringing the right clothes and shoes with you to work.

- craft the right soundtrack, and start listening to it just before it's time to work out.

- pick a mantra like *I got this!* and give yourself a mini pep-talk before your workouts.

Creating a Conducive Environment for Fitness at Work

Outside of your individual efforts, the landscape of your physical and social workplace can also mess with your ability to effectively transition.

For one thing, your office setup is likely not ideal when it comes to keeping you fit. Sitting all day is enough to take a toll on your health, but sitting with poor ergonomics compounds the problem and causes several adverse effects. The discomfort you feel when you sit for long periods may be due to things like an inadequate chair and desk height, improper keyboard or mouse placement, or poorly positioned monitors. Musculoskeletal discomfort over a sustained period of time can also cause repetitive strain injuries, or RSIs, like carpal tunnel syndrome, tendinitis, and other pain in the hands and wrists. If you're anything like me, staring at a computer all day can sometimes cause eye pain, especially if you already have worsening vision.

All of this can be adjusted with proper ergonomics, good lighting, and nice equipment, but there's ultimately no replacement for getting up and moving. During the workday, try to move as much as you can, even if it's just a quick stretch.

Incorporating Micro-Workouts Into the Workday

In the spirit of staving off a completely sedentary lifestyle, micro-workouts can boost your energy levels and decrease all of the aforementioned effects that come with working in a traditional office setting. While they're not a replacement for full workouts, micro-workouts can be a great option for those who don't have enough time or space to squeeze a workout into the workday.

The next time you're mulling over a big problem at work, try out some mini-workouts like:

- chair squats

- wall sits

- lunges

You should try to do as many reps as possible without overexerting yourself. After all, you don't want to go back to your desk exhausted! In Chapter 11, we'll explore a more in-depth office routine.

Cultivating a Fitness-Friendly Office Culture

While you don't necessarily have to go to an office-wide pilates class, there are a couple of things you can do to cultivate a fitness-forward attitude in your office. This isn't a top-down endeavor, either—leading by example works just as well as any other method, and this is something you might want to consider when talking about fitness at work.

Aside from doing your best on your own fitness journey, it's also important that you keep the welfare of your coworkers in mind. Suggesting regular movement breaks and designating specific *mini fitness* spaces in your office can create a more community-oriented approach to health. Group fitness activities can also be a great starting point as well. Fitness challenges, wellness programs, and educational opportunities like workshops can promote healthier working environments. This isn't just for your personal benefit, either. Fitness-friendly office cultures can

- lower overall healthcare costs.

- decrease absenteeism.

- decrease stress levels.

- enhance work performance.

- increase teamwork and camaraderie.

Now that you know the basics of the work-to-workout transition, it's time to focus on the content of your workouts. For professionals and busy self-starters, one thing is almost always at the forefront of your fitness journey: stress. In the next chapter, we'll discuss work-related stress, where it comes from, and how to bust through stressful times with exercise.

Chapter 3:

Stress-Busting Exercises for the Busy Professional

There are many sources of stress in the professional world, nearly too many to count. Adding the pressure of fitness onto the preexisting pile of work stress can sometimes feel like adding gas to a raging fire. But ultimately, fitness and daily workouts are in your best interests, both for long-term physical health and professional productivity. Just take it from Steven Branco, an entrepreneur, content creator, men's lifestyle writer, and expert on multitasking (Khoo, 2020):

> It's a love-hate relationship, for sure. Love the outcome, hate the process and how you feel in the moment. [I] definitely understand that the hard work will pay off. With such a high-stress job and sitting behind a laptop—in, most of the time, very non-ergonomically friendly ways—you get aches and pains. Working out helps deal with that. I wish I had more time [for fitness], but when you're hustling to achieve a dream, every minute counts. And when you're finally seeing the trajectory, it's easy to put yourself last to work toward your career goals.

Understanding the Relationship Between Exercise and Stress

Saying that fitness helps alleviate workplace stress is all well and good, but what do scientists and medical professionals say?

According to the Mayo Clinic, there are a number of ways that exercise, even in small amounts, can decrease your stress levels. This isn't just conjecture or opinion; your body responds to exercise with a number of measurable elements, making the scientific relationship between exercise and stress easy to spot. While science is finding new ways to explain this relationship every day, here's what we know about how exercise impacts your stress levels (Mayo Clinic Staff, 2022):

- Exercise increases endorphin levels. When you work out, your brain releases neurotransmitters called endorphins that make you feel good. This happens during any aerobic activity.

- It gets you thinking in the present moment. When you perform activities that are very physically engaging, you'll find all of your attention is devoted to what you're doing. This is doubly true if you enjoy the workout you're doing, like taking a nice hike or playing a great game of volleyball. When you stay in the moment like this, the worries from your professional life are usually quickly forgotten.

- It improves your overall mood. In numerous research studies, consistent exercise has been proven to lower symptoms of depression and anxiety significantly. While it's not a complete cure for symptoms of mental illness, working out can help stave off bouts of negative emotions and ailments.

Identifying Stress Triggers in a Professional Setting

For many of us, it often seems like work-related stress is endless. Sometimes, it feels like there are a million ways in which things can go wrong in your professional life, and this feeling takes a toll on your physical health. That being said, it can also be difficult to see major stressors coming, especially when everything seems fine on the surface. The best prevention measure in your arsenal is knowledge, so it's crucial to watch out for potential stressors like:

- a toxic workplace

- poor management

- job scope and demands

- physical work environment

- professional relationships

- lack of support

- role conflict

- harassment, discrimination, or trauma events

Any one of these things can turn into long-term stress that impacts your mental and physical health—not to mention your productivity.

Effective Stress-Busting Workouts

While science says that most forms of exercise can act as stress-relievers, there are several calming exercises you can turn to when you're feeling particularly stressed. This includes activities like:

- yoga

- tai chi

- pilates

- team sports

- martial arts

- outdoor activities

Slower, more intentional workouts like yoga and tai chi can also give you time to reflect and unwind during the time that you would otherwise spend sitting in front of the television or scrolling on social media. On other days, you might seek more intense activities like martial arts or team sports to distract you and take your mind off work. No matter what you choose, the important part is that you get your body moving!

Integrating Mindfulness Into Exercise

Mindfulness and exercise go hand-in-hand in many ways. When you're doing an activity that requires focus and attention to your body, it's more difficult for your mind to drift off. Elevating your exercise routine with intentional mindfulness transforms it into a holistic experience, enriching not only physical health but also mental and emotional well-being.

For those new to mindfulness, mindful breathing is a great place to start. The idea is relatively simple: Breathe slowly and deeply, allowing each inhale and exhale to guide your movements and center you in the present moment. Body scans are another great starting point—try to feel each part of your body, from your toes to the top of your head, one piece at a time. Whether walking, running, or doing yoga, channel mindfulness into each step, movement, and breath. Consciously focus on sounds, sensations, and your surroundings to deepen the mind-body connection.

Incorporating Stress-Busting Exercises Into a Busy Schedule

High-stress periods are often accompanied by additional responsibilities, worries, or to-dos at work. As a result, your schedule may get busier, and you may find yourself at a loss in terms of integrating workouts into your schedule. During these times, it's important to take it easy on yourself to prevent burnout. If there's absolutely no way that you can get in a 30-minute workout, there are still some steps you can take to avoid falling off the wagon completely.

Quick and Effective Stress-Relief Exercises for the Office

While you may not feel comfortable doing lunges in the middle of the office during a stressful workday, you can still take a few minutes every now and then to decompress and center yourself.

They might not be HIIT-worthy exercises, but these are still some good tools to keep in your metaphorical toolbox during stressful times:

- deep breathing

- light stretching

- shoulder rolls

- desk push-ups

- stress ball squeezes

- seated torso twists

Making Time for Regular Stress-Relief Workouts

Ultimately, there will come a time when you have to choose between fitness and other important aspects of your life. This is when carving out 30 minutes per day starts getting tricky. If you're truly committed to your long-term health, you'll find a way to make it happen. This is something that Palak Loizides, CEO of Embiria, has experienced firsthand (Khoo, 2020):

> [I value fitness] so much so that I'll make time for it—even if that means waking up at 6:30 a.m. to get a class in—and I am typically not a morning person. You make time for whatever is a priority to you.

It won't always be easy—frankly, sticking to your fitness goals will probably be difficult at times. But, in the end, your physical health, mental well-being, and professional productivity will thank you if you take care of your body.

Combining Physical Activity With Other Stress Management Techniques

Of course, fighting stress is more than just exercising the anxiety away. Here, fitness is one piece of a larger self-care puzzle. Other crucial pieces include aspects of mental healthcare, such as therapy, journaling, and keeping a healthy social life. When things get difficult, you can use your fitness goals in conjunction with other self-care methods to create an even more potent antidote to work-related stress. The next time you find yourself in a stressful mentality, try taking a long, hot shower after your stress-busting workout.

Maximizing the Mental Benefits of Exercise

To explore the mental benefits of exercise, let's go back to Palak Loizides (Khoo, 2020):

> Losing weight and staying fit used to be my main priority, but now I do it because of so much more than that. I value being able to move my body more easily, making healthier food choices, and building strength and resilience both physically and emotionally.

According to research, fitness does much more than just keep you in shape. People who exercise regularly have been shown to have better mental health outcomes, better interpersonal relationships—and more of them—a better self-image, and far lower rates of mental illness. Additionally, this relationship works the other way around; with better mental health outcomes, you're more likely to want to better yourself and stick to your fitness goals.

So far, we've mostly talked about the preparation and content of your workouts. There's one thing we haven't yet discussed, and it's integral to redefining fitness as we know it. Your workout setting, despite what you may have been led to believe by social media, isn't limited to just the gym. In the next chapter, we'll explore some fun and efficient alternatives to getting a gym membership.

Chapter 4:

The No-Gym-Required Routine

Instead of trying to convince you myself, I'll let one busy professional tell you themself. Doctors are perhaps some of the most busy people in the professional world, and their line of work requires immense physical and mental energy for long hours. According to one doctor—Dr. Tello—however, that shouldn't stop anyone from sneaking fitness into their day (2017):

> Today, I led a small group of medical students on inpatient rounds. We had a patient on the 7th floor of the hospital. As I always do, I headed for the stairs but told the students they could take the elevators if they wanted—I promised them that they wouldn't lose any points on their academic performance! And as they usually do, they decided to join me in the stairwell. Yes, we huffed and puffed a bit, but we still chatted, discussing fitness the whole time. I take the stairs for many reasons... but a bigger factor is my own vigorous, unapologetic self-care regimen. I know I need regular exercise to maintain my mood and my health, so I fit it in wherever I can. If I have a patient on the 7th floor—or even the 22nd floor—I look at it as a terrific opportunity for a mini-workout in the middle of my workday.

Embracing the Flexibility of No-Gym Workouts

As we saw above, no time or place is set in stone when it comes to fitness. Rather, professionals who are committed to fitness find many different ways to stay fit, oftentimes outside of the gym. This fluidity in approach can lead you to a far more sustainable and comprehensive idea of fitness than you'd find in a traditional gym setting. While there are no hard and fast rules about where to do your workouts, it's worth considering alternative settings in place of the traditional gym.

Advantages of No-Gym Workouts

Gyms certainly have a variety of benefits to offer patrons—fancy machinery to work every muscle, access to classes, and other amenities you won't find anywhere else. That being said, it's not all about machines. There are several benefits to skipping a gym membership, including:

- Convenience and affordability: When fitness isn't limited to a specific place, it effectively frees you up to get a workout anywhere you can. Logistically, that's less time, energy, and money spent on getting from work to the gym every day. Instead of worrying about finding the right gym or paying for an expensive membership, all you have to do is find the nearest public park or open area.

- Adjustability by fitness level: As we've touched on before, gyms can sometimes be intimidating for beginners. If you don't know how to use equipment or feel self-conscious about how you look, an at-home workout can be a great intro to the world of fitness. On the opposite end of the spectrum, at-home workouts and outdoor workouts can still be altered depending on how experienced you are.

- Emphasizing the basics: Rather than prompting you to buy fancy—and usually expensive—workout equipment or tools, a lot of routines for alternative workout settings emphasize going back to the basics. At-home machines may be nice to have, but all you really need is an open space to work with.

Overcoming the Mindset of Needing a Gym

If you're anything like me, you probably dreaded fitness exams in school. My least favorite exam was the pacer, a timed exercise that progressed from walking to sprinting over the course of about half an hour. The running wasn't the most difficult part—it was running in a gym full of peers who would see my score, dependent on which stage of the exercise I failed. It took me a while to overcome the traumatizing—and mostly embarrassing—memory of the pacer, but when I did, I suddenly realized that I loved running! I was suddenly exercising consistently, despite the memory of the pacer exam. Crucially, I discovered that exercising outside of the gym could be a lot more fulfilling—and a lot less nerve-wracking—than trekking to the gym every day while still accomplishing the same goals.

As an adult, the anxiety that accompanies going to a gym can feel a bit like the pacer did in grade school; potentially failing in a room full of peers is deeply discouraging for many people. Not exercising isn't an option, however. The middle ground—no-gym workouts—is a great starting place for those who feel uncertain about getting a gym membership. Despite what we see on social media, fitness isn't tied to a specific place or time. Fitness is a lifestyle choice, one that can thrive both in and outside of a traditional gym setting—as long as we commit ourselves to the choice.

Setting Realistic Expectations

The relationship between expectations and goals can be a tricky one to navigate, especially considering all of the glamorized fitness content we see online. Deconstructing our expectations of ourselves and our bodies—which are often far too high—takes a lot of mental work, and it can sometimes be disheartening to see the difference between where we are and where we want to be.

The best way to deconstruct our expectations is to measure where we currently fall. Establishing a general fitness baseline can be accomplished by testing areas of your body periodically through things like:

- testing cardiovascular endurance through tests like the pacer

- testing muscular strength by performing drills or reps

- measuring metrics like weight, body fat percentage, and resting heart rate

When you examine these metrics, be sure to record your findings in some way, like a fitness journal or digital documentation.

Designing Effective No-Gym Workouts

The combination of no-gym exercises and your ability to create routines can make for an excellent long-term skill when it comes to fitness. This key tenet allows you to free yourself from the walls of a gym and make fitness a bigger and more meaningful element of your life. To do this, there are two things to remember when designing no-gym routines: bodyweight training and HIIT.

Fundamentals of Bodyweight Training

One of the most important aspects of no-gym routines is bodyweight exercising. Traditional gyms often minimize bodyweight exercises in favor of adding additional weight without changing form, like putting weights on a bar while doing squats. Bodyweight training effectively does the opposite, changing form and using physics to increase the intensity of your exercise. This is also known as resistance exercise because it relies on the resistance provided by your own body weight.

This is an extremely versatile and effective way to build strength, endurance, and flexibility without the need for external equipment. Basic exercises include things like squats, lunges, and planks. These types of exercises leverage the natural movements of the body to engage multiple sets of muscle fibers, which in turn promotes strength in practical areas. Bodyweight training is accessible to all fitness levels, as it allows for modifications to intensity and complexity—think knee push-ups instead of normal push-ups.

Incorporating High-Intensity Interval Training (HIIT)

Bodyweight HIIT combines the efficiency of interval training with the effectiveness of bodyweight exercises to create a dynamic, intense, and accessible workout routine. Bodyweight HIIT routines typically include exercises like:

- burpees

- jumping jacks

- mountain climbers

- squat jumps

These exercises also engage several different sets of muscle groups simultaneously, and the intensity and rapidity of bodyweight exercises in an HIIT format can be just as good as running. This approach not only saves you the time of going to the gym, but it also enhances post-exercise calorie expenditure, known as the afterburn effect. In Chapter 11, we'll go over some specific routines you can use in various locations.

Another issue arises, however, when busy professionals try to set aside time for longer workouts. Even when you don't need any equipment or a gym to work out, getting 30 minutes of exercise on the books consistently can be a struggle. In the next chapter, we'll talk about some methods you can use to effectively schedule your fitness routines and prioritize your health in the face of busy schedules.

Chapter 5:

Scheduling Fitness Into Your Work Calendar

Usually, the phrase *no time* doesn't actually indicate a fully packed schedule. Rather, we use this to talk about how much mental or physical energy we'll have after whatever is on our plate at work. In truth, this is a question of time management, which is something you'll have to master in order to achieve long-term results in your fitness journey. According to businesswoman and entrepreneur Nikki Bettilini (Khoo, 2020):

> It's made me much more scheduled. Before owning my own business, I would work out when I could fit it in and didn't really have a plan or a schedule. Now, I know that working out helps my mental health and makes me more productive, so I make a point to schedule my workouts into my calendar to make sure I don't miss them. Currently, I'm finding that 5 p.m. workouts are best for my schedule, but the days vary based on meetings and events.

You'll never really have *enough* time or energy to properly dedicate yourself to your fitness. Knowing this, it's even more important to try your best to workout consistently, even if it means choosing to prioritize fitness over other comparable things.

Understanding the Importance of Scheduling Exercise

This all comes down to scheduling. I don't know about you, but when I'm exhausted or bored, I tend to stick to the easiest schedule I can get my hands on. If you don't feel like you have the energy to work out, you probably won't have the energy to schedule your fitness in the moment. The key here is to plan ahead.

The Role of Planning in Fitness Success

Planning and scheduling in advance play crucial roles in achieving fitness success by providing structure, consistency, and a roadmap for progress. A well-thought-out fitness plan will help you define specific goals and stick to your routines, even when you're feeling stressed or tired. Scheduling workouts into a weekly or monthly routine creates a commitment to regular exercise, making it a priority in busy schedules.

Out of all of this, consistency is perhaps the biggest aspect of planning that will help you in the long run. A planned schedule ensures that your workouts become a regular part of your routine, reducing the likelihood of skipping sessions. Scheduling in advance also allows for a more balanced and well-rounded workout, rather than just doing whatever you feel like at the moment.

If you have a consistent routine on the books, you'll also be able to track your progress over time, meeting your fitness goals in an even, timely manner.

Time Management for Busy Professionals

In Chapter 1, we talked a little bit about time confetti and intentional exercise. Luckily for busy professionals, this is just one scheduling technique—here, we'll take a look at several more:

- Organize your activities based on natural energy levels: Are you more of an early bird or a night owl? If you're a morning person, trying to work out after a long day at work might be a little difficult. Alternatively, night owls will probably have more trouble waking up early over time. To make the most of your natural rhythms, make sure to schedule your workouts at times when you know you'll be more energized—or, at the very least, less tired.

- Daily planning: In addition to weekly and long-term planning of your routines, a quick five-minute once-over of your schedule on a particular day can give you an idea of what to look forward to when you work out. In addition to your basic routine for the day, you might also want to add exercises based on how your body feels.

- Prioritization: At some point, you'll have to prioritize your workouts over other things. This will probably feel terrible at first like you're shirking responsibility or using fitness to get away from other obligations. In reality, prioritizing fitness is just giving back to yourself, which, in turn, will prepare you for all your other responsibilities.

- Outsourcing when possible: If possible, make your schedule a little less hectic by outsourcing some of the easier tasks on your to-do. For instance, if you have the resources, think about hiring a cleaner for your household chores.

- Minimize distractions as much as possible: When we see work notifications pop up on our phones when we're not at work, we often feel obligated to jump into action. In truth, there are very few work tasks that can't wait. Even if it makes you feel lazy, try to keep the work notifications at bay as best as you can by turning off your notifications when you work out.

- Deconstruct your idea of *done*: If you're a high-achiever or a perfectionist, you may have trouble finishing tasks if they're not up to your standards. In fitness, this approach rarely works, and it will more than likely land you in the realm of overtraining. When you transition from work to workout, consider it a transition from the perfectionist side of your brain to its self-care side.

Strategies for Incorporating Exercise Into the Workday

In previous chapters, we've talked a bit about things like micro-workouts that help you get some extra movement in during the workday, as well as other methods like biking or running to the office. That being said, these things may not scratch the itch that you have for a full workout. If this sounds like you, then it's important to find ways to incorporate full workouts into your workday. To do this, calendar-blocking will be your best friend.

Leveraging Technology for Scheduling and Reminders

The number of fitness apps currently on the market is truly astounding. According to one survey by Straits Research, there are a whopping 97,000 different fitness and wellness apps on the IOS and Android App Store, not including built-in features like Samsung Health (Straits Research, 2021). With the sheer size of this area of the market, choosing which app to use can be a daunting task.

On the bright side, a corner of this market specializes in fitness scheduling. That is, these apps focus on fitting your workouts into your schedule rather than giving you complete workout routines to do. While there are several hundred different options to choose from, here are some good starting places for beginners:

- Mindbody

- Jefit

- Fitnotes

- Fitbod

Once you've found software that you like, it's time to do the hard stuff: blocking your calendar. When you sit down to block your calendar, don't leave any room for work to creep in. To the best of your ability, try not to make your daily workout negotiable in the face of menial workplace tasks.

Creating a Consistent Workout Routine

As you may have noticed, consistency is key to long-term success. You'll be far less likely to ditch your workout plan entirely if you have a plan on the books—literally, written down and placed somewhere visible. During times when the consistency of your workouts might be in danger, it's crucial to look at the bigger picture of what you're hoping to achieve. For this purpose, goal-setting can rescue a workout plan at risk of abandonment.

Setting Short- and Long-Term Fitness Goals

In the last chapter, we talked a bit about setting realistic expectations. Whether you use a gym or not, expectations are an important aspect of long-term planning. When considering your fitness schedule, it's crucial that you look at both the short- and long-term goals you have in mind, as well as the metrics you'll need to reach to get there. These will ultimately depend on the baseline you established in the last chapter, and your goals will generally aim to improve these metrics.

The idea of metrics is part of a larger picture when it comes to setting goals. You've likely heard of the SMART method of goal-setting, which includes elements that are:

- **S**pecific: Stating what needs to happen and how you're going to do it in full detail.

- **M**easurable: Quantifying your goals through metrics, numbers, and benchmarks.

- **A**chievable: Reaching just outside of your comfort zone—but not quite shooting for the stars.

- **R**elevant: Staying on track by revolving around your broader health goals.

- **T**ime-based: When exactly you're going to meet your goals.

Oftentimes, it can be very helpful to write your short- and long-term goals down somewhere special, like a Google Doc or a physical journal. Your short-term goals might look something like this:

For the next two weeks, I am going to add an extra five reps of push-ups to each of my workouts.

A good long-term goal might look something like this:

By the end of the year, I will be able to run a seven-minute mile.

Accountability and Support Systems

There's a reason why hitting the gym is such a popular New Year's resolution: Many folks who want to get into fitness aspire to go to the gym, then eventually fall off the wagon by the next New Year. One examination of this phenomenon concluded that fitness resolutions were given up as early as mid-January, meaning that the life expectancy of fitness goals was only about two weeks on average (Poon, 2019).

At this point, we know that fitness is a lifestyle choice, not a one-time vacation into cardio or weightlifting. Luckily, we've already covered the first two steps that will prevent you from falling off the wagon: awareness of potential pitfalls and recording your goals. Sometimes, however, these two things aren't enough to keep you on track. If you're anxious about staying up on your workout routine, try a few of these methods:

- Post your goals on social media—if you have personal social media accounts—or tell your friends and family about your fitness goals.

- Sign up for group events with other people, either by yourself or with friends.

- Celebrate your milestones with small treats that motivate you.

Flexible Scheduling for Unpredictable Workdays

Steven Branco, businessman and content creator, has some thoughts about this area. In one interview, Branco states (Khoo, 2020):

> Being so busy, it's hard to build consistency, which is what I feel is necessary to really get a workout regimen going. Both as an entrepreneur and as a writer and editor, they're both very demanding roles, so it's tough. I don't want to [restrain] myself to not have any time for fitness because I know how important it is. So, I just try to fit in any form of extra activity and steps as possible. Heck, you might even catch me doing lunges up or down [Toronto's] Yonge Street on my way home from work!

When your workout routine feels like it's in jeopardy due to unforeseen and unavoidable scheduling conflicts, consider making your idea of fitness more flexible. Rather than ditching your fitness efforts altogether when things get busy, try to get in as much activity as you can in the form of everyday tasks.

Another key aspect of scheduling is nutrition. Aside from physical activity, what you eat is one of the most important parts of staying fit. Scheduling time to cook, buy groceries, and eat, however, can be even more difficult than working out. In the next chapter, we'll go over some key parts of nutrition, including meal preparation, scheduling, and a couple of kitchen hacks to save you time.

Chapter 6:

Nutrition for the Time-Pressed

When you stop and think about it, your body is always *on*—keeping you breathing, pumping blood around your body, and releasing neurochemicals that instruct your cells what to do to keep you alive. For business people with packed schedules, there's no real *off* switch. This can sometimes feel like a curse instead of a blessing, especially when our schedules get so packed that we feel suffocated.

Given that your body never truly rests all at once, it's crucial that you fuel it with the right things. Eating high-quality foods with the proper nutrients, vitamins, and minerals can keep you going, even through the most stressful of workdays.

Understanding the Link Between Nutrition and Fitness

Fitness is a relatively high-cost activity when it comes to the metaphorical fuel your body needs to live. You burn more calories sprinting than you do sitting still, which makes the fuel that you burn even more important. Unfortunately, it's easy to fuel your body with the wrong kinds of energy. Food high in refined sugars, for instance, has been proven to be harmful to the brain, with effects such as:

- worsening your body's insulin response

- promoting inflammation

- increasing oxidative stress levels

- increasing the likelihood of moodiness, diagnosable mood disorders, and depression

In fact, high levels of refined sugars have even been proven to cause mental impairment and worse cognitive functions (Selhub, 2022). Unfortunately, refined sugar is just one element of a bad diet—in our world today, there are several *fuel* options that actually make it harder for our bodies to work effectively. If you want your fitness journey to last, it's crucial that you understand the basics of a good diet.

The Role of Nutrition in Achieving Fitness Goals

The different parts of your body, while needing the same general energy, process energy in different ways. For instance, you probably know that protein is an important nutrient for building muscle, whereas carrots are supposedly good for the eyes. Much of what you hear on this front is old wives' tales, but there is some truth to the idea that our bodies process different food items differently.

Within the scope of physical fitness, there are a of couple areas that you want to pay attention to generally, including bone strength, muscles, and brain function. Your muscles, for instance, break down protein in a process called muscle protein synthesis. In general terms, it works something like this: You eat a source of protein, like chicken, and your gut gets to work digesting everything by sending nutrients to different parts of your body. When your muscle cells get their dose of protein, they effectively use that protein to rebuild themselves, which in turn builds muscle mass, repairs cellular muscle damage from workouts, and makes you stronger. This is why you'll often hear fitness enthusiasts and nutritionists emphasize the importance of protein sources in your diet.

Protein, while important, is just one aspect of your diet. There are dozens of other elements like macronutrients—carbohydrates, proteins, and fats—and micronutrients—vitamins and minerals—that work to keep your body healthy and happy.

Basic Principles of a Healthy Diet for Busy Individuals

Online, there is *a lot* of content when it comes to nutrition and fitness. In addition to the wide expanse of knowledge out there, there are also a lot of opinions and disinformation, especially from those who claim to be certified nutritionists. In short, the Google search box—and social media platforms like Instagram, in particular—is a minefield littered with ads, fad products, and potentially harmful practices.

When exploring nutrition advice online, it's extremely important to exercise caution. As a general rule, it's paramount that you run any new diets, foods, or routines by your doctor before you try to adopt them into your lifestyle. That goes for the contents of this book as well—when in doubt, talk to your doctor!

When we set aside the fads and bad information, though, there are a couple of key principles that emerge:

- Water is essential: Instead of drinking sodas, alcohol, or even carbonated waters, plain old still water will always be your best bet when it comes to physical health.

- Avoiding processed foods: The occasional protein bar won't hurt you too much, but whole foods like fruits and veggies are the superior option.

- More is less: You may be tempted to cut down on your portion sizes when you think about nutrition. However, the amount of food you eat won't make much of a difference if the quality of food you eat is poor. Before you start skipping breakfast, try adjusting the content of your breakfasts first.

- Meals are a balancing act: When you were in school, you might've been taught about the food pyramid published by the U.S. government. This may be a great place to start thinking about food groups and meal composition, but it's certainly not the end-all-be-all. In general, you should listen to what your body tells you to eat; if you want bread, reach for the sourdough. That being said, more fruits, veggies, and whole grains are usually a safe bet when you're at a loss for how to balance your meals.

Quick and Healthy Meal Ideas

The concept of meal-prepping isn't new—for much of human history, we've been preserving food through drying, canning, or pickling processes. Meal-prepping is the modern-day answer to packed schedules and limited resources. The idea behind meal-prepping is relatively simple: Once per week, take a few hours to prepare, cook, and package meals so you can save time later in the week. This is a great tool for busy professionals, even if you're not the best cook.

Efficient Meal Preparation Strategies

At first glance, meal-prepping can be overwhelming for beginners. Even for experienced meal-preppers, the prospect of scheduling, buying ingredients, cooking, and storing can become a cumbersome task that takes up space on your to-do list. However, if done right, meal-prepping can save you a lot of time throughout the week.

Whether you're new to meal-prepping or you've done it for years, here are a couple of things to keep in mind while you prepare:

- Make a plan. Like with fitness, you'll want to brainstorm and write down a plan before you try to do anything new. This usually means doing some research online or asking friends and family for easy recipes that can be frozen and reheated.

- Take stock and organize your pantry—if you have one. Before you go grocery shopping, you need to know what you have. When possible—and when it's safe to do so—try to use as much of what you already have instead of buying brand-new ingredients.

- Keep it in season. When you're grocery shopping for fresh, whole, unprocessed foods, you're likely to encounter some constraints. The biggest of these is seasonal restrictions, which can make shopping for out-of-season goods difficult. To save you time and energy, try to stick to recipes that use seasonal ingredients.

- Make good use of spices and herbs. Prepackaged meals can get very boring very fast. When you're in need of some extra oomph for your day, try including spices and herbs in your recipes.

- Keep it simple and consider the essentials. If you're a beginner, you may be tempted to dive head-first into cooking and trying out new meals. While this is okay sometimes, it's important not to overcomplicate things too much.

Supplements and Their Role

If you thought nutrition misinformation was bad, you'll probably be less than thrilled to learn about the dietary supplement industry. Unfortunately, dietary supplements in the US are not nearly as regulated as food or drugs—even the products you purchase in brick-and-mortar stores like Trader Joe's aren't always truthful in their advertising.

Take Ephedra, a popular weight loss supplement that made the rounds a few years ago. Ephedra, despite being sold in traditional stores, was later linked to a series of sudden deaths and nasty side effects, according to Harvard Health Publishing. To make matters worse for consumers, even seemingly safe supplements like Iron or vitamin B can contain unsafe levels of vitamins and minerals. For instance, taken at levels higher than 2.4 mg per day, vitamin B can cause headaches, nausea, vomiting, fatigue, and tingling in the extremities. Additionally, recent studies have shown that dietary supplements aren't especially effective at staving off illnesses—like the common cold treatment of vitamin C supplements. Given that Americans spend over $25 billion per year on supplements, these side effects have the potential to be wide-reaching

(Skerret, 2012). Furthermore, some manufacturers can get away with using poor-quality or even harmful ingredients in their products. This makes it doubly important to check the labels on any supplements you're considering for purchase.

With ineffective results at best and adverse results at worst, the world of over-the-counter supplements is tricky to navigate, even for the most well-versed fitness enthusiast. In turn, this makes research and self-education on supplements *absolutely necessary* before incorporating anything new into your diet. Moreover, your general practitioner will likely have some great insights into what supplements are dangerous, ineffective, or wrong for you. This is especially true for those who are on medications like blood thinners, which can interact negatively with supplements like vitamin K. In short, talk to your doctor!

That being said, supplements certainly play an important role for some. Supplements with good ingredients and proper levels of nutrients can be a great addition to your diet. With supplements, your goal should ultimately be to fill in the gaps in your diet. To do this, you should have a working knowledge of what micro and macronutrients your diet lacks. Yet again, talking to your doctor is very helpful with this. Nevertheless, there are a couple of common areas where American diets are lacking (*Office of Dietary Supplements*, 2020), including:

- calcium

- vitamins D, C, and E

- folic acid—particularly for women

- omega-3 fatty acids

- zinc, copper, and lutein

When shopping for supplements like the ones above, make sure to look at the amount of each dosage—the dosage should align with the daily recommended vitamin and mineral intake, as prescribed by the National Institutes of Health.

Balancing Nutrition With a Hectic Lifestyle

When it comes to busy lifestyles, nutrition can sometimes be a source of stress. You could spend hours looking at tasty videos from Buzzfeed or kitchen hacks on Instagram Reels. Social media isn't necessarily a bad source of diet inspiration—though multiple hours online might be a little much. For beginners, however, a lot of what you might see online can feel unattainable. Like workout routines, we have to temper our expectations when we examine online food and nutrition content.

While Reels with perfectly baked sourdough and dazzlingly grilled veggies are certainly pretty to look at, there's really no substitute for good old-fashioned kitchen know-how. Whether you're a novice or a pro home chef, it's always worth going back to the basics. Some key tenets of home cooking include:

- keeping a clean, organized workspace

- writing down the keepers in a recipe book

- making good use of your freezer

- mise en place, or getting all of your preparation out of the way before you start constructing a meal

Integrating Healthy Eating Into Daily Routines

Healthy eating can be tough, especially if you're traveling. Every fast food sign turns into an advertisement that essentially trades your health and wellness for convenience and affordability. Effective meal-prepping cuts out this temptation completely. Even if you're not the greatest chef, there are still delicious, time-efficient, nutritious meals that you can prepare as a beginner. To help you make the most out of your meal plans, let's take a look at some things you can incorporate into your weekly preparations:

- The one-pan plan minimizes dishes used and saves you the trouble of washing dishes later.

- Experiment with new proteins, like seafood or dairy—if your health allows.

- Mix and match by preparing smaller sides and having a tapas-like meal.

- When in doubt, blend together some fruits and veggies to make an on-the-go smoothie.

- Jack-of-all-foods and superfoods, such as cauliflower, chia seeds, and Greek yogurt.

Social Eating and Maintaining Dietary Goals

Sometimes, eating is akin to other vices like smoking or drinking. Fast and easily affordable food that you might find in most places is often packed with sugar, fat, carbs, preservatives, and other processed junk. Unfortunately for us, our bodies are basically wired to cram as many tasty calories into them as possible, even if it's not good for us. Like the occasional drink, a drive-through meal won't kill you or derail your fitness goals. But, in excess, poor food choices can take a toll on your body.

When you're enjoying an indulgent meal with friends or family, less-than-nutritious foods pose a double threat. In addition to straying from your fitness goals, it can also feel like you're being forced to eat poorly in order to enjoy yourself. From birthday parties to holidays, there's a lot of room for bad nutrition choices. To combat this, here are a couple of things to keep in mind at your next food-based gathering:

- Don't go anywhere hungry.

- Only fill the tank to 80%.

- Try to physically move away from the food area.

- Socialize.

- Drink water.

- Eat slowly.

Ultimately, despite our best efforts, we all fall prey to a fatty, sugary, carb-filled treat every now and again. If we didn't, we wouldn't be human! When these things happen, try not to penalize yourself too much. Keep the negative self-talk at bay by remembering your achievements, and don't punish yourself with extra sprints the next day. Guilt won't keep you on track in the long run, but it will surely ruin your mental health. If, every once in a blue moon, you're really, *really* craving a burger—and you've tried your best to stay on track—there's nothing to do but indulge.

In these instances, substitution might be a good option to avoid falling off the wagon. A traditional burger, for example, might be replaced with a lettuce-wrapped burger, skipping the bun. You may also want to try skipping the sauces, as these are normally high in sodium and sugar.

Chapter 7:

Short Workouts, Long-Term Results

Sustainability is often an elusive animal, especially in today's day and age of instant gratification. You don't want your fitness journey to feel like a stop-and-start mission, giving in to the pressures of the outside world. Instead, true fitness requires us to find ways of making our workouts sustainable, ideally over several decades. To do this, workout design also needs to keep sustainability in mind.

The Efficacy of Short Workouts

In Chapter 1, we discussed some of the short-term reasons why routines like HIIT are more efficient than other fitness frameworks. In addition to being a good short-term choice, both for your valuable time and your fitness goals, there is actually scientific evidence that suggests HIIT is more impactful in the long run.

The Science Behind Short-Duration Exercise

According to one research study, participants who performed HIIT routines for a sustained period of 12 weeks experienced a 27% higher aerobic capacity than the control group. Furthermore, participants in the study group—those on a HIIT program—saw higher glycogen concentrations and lower physiological stress after a long-term routine (Araujo et al., 2016). The 3 key terms here are *aerobic capacity*, *glycogen concentrations*, and *physiological stress*.

Let's start with aerobic capacity. You may remember our definition of intensity in exercise from Chapter 1—in short, how close to your maximum heart rate you get as you perform an exercise. High-intensity exercises mean a higher heart rate, while low-intensity exercises mean a lower heart rate. Aerobic capacity runs parallel to this idea, but the concept of aerobic capacity comes a little bit closer to the scientific truth. When you do aerobic exercise like cardio, your body uses up oxygen to let you keep moving. By extension, higher oxygen levels in your blood result in a better ability to continue moving freely. A higher aerobic capacity therefore means that your blood can carry more oxygen during intense exercise, allowing you to operate at high levels of intensity for longer.

Next, let's look at glycogen concentrations, specifically in muscle. This sounds like a complicated term, so let's break it down a little bit. When you eat carbohydrates, your body breaks them down into sugar molecules called glucose. Glucose needs to be stored when it isn't used, so your body turns it into glycogen until you need energy. Glycogen is stored in two places in your body: the liver and the muscles. The tiny glycogen clusters in your muscles act like mini snacks—for these muscles—which can be very helpful when they're doing a lot of intense work. In other words, higher muscle glycogen means that your muscles have an energy source at the ready, so they're more prepared to work hard when needed.

Finally, physiological stress is essentially a physical manifestation of mental or emotional stress you carry. This physical stress can result in markers that scientists can quantitatively measure over time, like cortisol—often called the stress hormone. Having too many of these markers in your body in the long term can result in adverse effects like fatigue, fitness plateau, and even other mental effects like depression or anxiety. So, lower amounts of stress markers in the body ultimately mean being happier and healthier.

In other words, short workouts like HIIT can massively impact the physical and mental benefits you see as you progress on your workout journey.

Designing Effective Short Workout Routines

Knowing all of this, how can you design workouts that rise to the challenges of competing attention, long-term sustainability, and joy? All of these factors are tricky to take into account, but crafting a good workout routine is still entirely within reach. By knowing a couple of the basics of workout design, you can create a routine that will last for years—while still being fun to do.

Principles of Efficient Workout Design

We've gone over several different workouts in the previous chapters, but there are dozens more that you can integrate into your daily fitness regimen. Furthermore, there are just about a million different ways that you can put everything together. It's a little overwhelming at first, which is perhaps why so many beginners turn to apps or online resources for help. Over time, though, you'll start wanting to customize your workouts to your specific needs, either through adjusting an existing workout plan or building your own from scratch.

No matter where you fall on the spectrum, it's a good idea to think about how your workouts are constructed. To do this, consider a couple of guidelines for designing optimal workouts:

- What are your current goals?

- What workout location is best for you?

- What is the simplest way to target your focus areas?

Sustaining Long-Term Health and Fitness

Long-term fitness requires workouts that will follow you throughout the years, through periods of sickness, aging, and other big life events. You'll need to periodically reassess your workouts, their effectiveness, and your progress using the metrics we discussed back in Chapters 1 and 2. Additionally, it's a good idea to have methods of tracking your long-term progress in your back pocket.

Tracking Progress Over Time

Over time, you'll find that tracking your progress is just as important as preparing and performing your workouts. This is partly the same reason why to-do lists feel so satisfying once you complete them—it's evidence of your accomplishments. No matter how small or insignificant they feel in the moment, each rep and each mile contribute to your health.

We've already touched on a couple of ways to track your short and long-term progress, but let's examine a couple of methods further:

- Keep a journal, either physical or virtual, that details the content of your daily workouts, how you feel about doing them, and what progress you're seeing.

- Take pictures to show to your future self.

- Be unconventional, like using your old clothes to see how far you've come.

- Use metrics—sparingly—like weight and BMI.

Overcoming Plateaus and Maintaining Motivation

Over long periods of time, you may find that motivation is difficult to maintain. There are several ways to combat this, including more accessible workouts, enjoyable exercises, and other motivating rewards. Erin Bury, cofounder and CEO of Willfull, describes her methods of motivation when it comes to long-term fitness (Khoo, 2020):

> Between my Barry's packages and ClassPass, I spend hundreds of dollars a month on fitness. It's my one luxury as a startup founder, and I believe it does have a huge positive impact on the business, so I can justify it.

Identifying and Overcoming Plateaus

Plateaus are perhaps the most disheartening experience for people of all levels. After a while, you'll start to notice that you're not making as much progress as you previously were. Despite your best efforts, the plateau might even persist over a period of weeks, making you feel frustrated. After all, progress doesn't feel nearly as good when you start thinking it's all futile. Even for the most experienced gym-goer, hitting this kind of wall can feel like a reason to stop working out altogether.

Plateaus happen for a number of reasons, but they're most commonly due to factors like:

- ineffective training routines for your level

- not pushing yourself enough

- inconsistent training

- a poor diet or lifestyle

- lack of sleep or poor quality of sleep

These factors already impact health in a big way, so the combination of direct effects and fitness plateaus is like a one-two punch of discouragement. Let's pause for a moment and recognize that keeping fit, no matter how small or futile it feels, is never a bad thing. Hitting stubborn plateaus, however crappy it feels, is just a part of long-term fitness that you'll have to overcome, both mentally and physically. To do so, you need to first equip yourself with more detailed knowledge about what a plateau might look like. Often, plateaus present with stagnation of weight loss, loss in muscle tone–mass, a general feeling of fatigue, and low motivation. In short, you'll feel pretty bad, but you won't necessarily be able to point to a specific reason why.

Luckily, there are a couple of steps you can take to fight fitness plateaus, even sometimes before they strike. This includes things like:

- changing your routine

- trying something new

- considering periodization training

- embracing progressive overload methods

- prioritizing recovery

Long-term fitness can be a tough thing to manage, but it will ultimately enrich your life. As a busy professional, however, you may often face challenges that don't affect other fitness enthusiasts. One facet of this is frequent travel, which can seem to blow a hole in your fitness routines... at first glance. In the next chapter, we'll cover fitness sustainability practices that you can use while on the road—or in the air.

Chapter 8

Workout Plans for the Frequent Traveler

Traveling, especially long-distance traveling, can feel like something of a workout in and of itself. The mental energy you use to adjust to constantly-changing surroundings, the physical energy you use to walk around to find gates and stations, and the emotional exhaustion of stress can all contribute to an overwhelming sense of tiredness. However, as we've seen, exercise can actually boost your energy levels and decrease stress, provided it's done right. This is invaluable when you're traveling, overcoming jetlag, and adjusting to new places.

Understanding the Challenges of Maintaining Fitness While Traveling

Staying committed to your fitness goals during travel poses several challenges, many of which might not even be on your radar. As always, the first step in overcoming these challenges is identifying what they are and then slowly working through them at whatever pace feels comfortable.

Identifying Common Obstacles for Travelers

According to Joe Muller—a digital nomad, fitness enthusiast, and writer for Freaking Nomads—there are several hurdles that travelers have to face when sticking to a consistent workout routine. While it's certainly possible, frequent fliers have to deal with things like:

- long hours, many of which are spent awake and alert for streams of new information

- irregular routines, which can mess with their natural rhythms and throw them off of your fitness game

- unfamiliar environments, where they might not always know where exactly to go for fitness purposes

In addition to these challenges of deprivation, travel also poses challenges of a different nature. Things like delicious food you've never tried and lounging around the hotel can also pull you away from your fitness goals. This is where the international McDonald's craze comes from, particularly when it comes to regional menus around the world. After all, who wouldn't want to try a squid ink burger when in Japan? While immersing yourself in your location and learning about local cultures is fantastic, be aware of some of the more sneaky pitfalls that can creep up on you.

The Importance of Staying Fit While Traveling

Staying fit while traveling is crucial for counteracting the sedentary nature of journeys, supporting physical and mental health, and enhancing the overall travel experience. Regular exercise helps combat stiffness from prolonged periods of inactivity, boosts the immune system, manages your stress, and contributes to stable and sustainable energy levels. It also provides a sense of routine amid the unpredictability of travel, further allowing for exploration of new landscapes when your energy levels allow. Ultimately, staying fit while on the road positively influences your well-being at a time when your body is more vulnerable than usual, making the travel experience enjoyable, energized, and healthy.

Setting Realistic Fitness Goals for Travel

While your rational mind knows the importance of fitness, there may still be unforeseen hurdles you haven't accounted for yet. This is the nature of travel, and unfortunately, for busy professionals, there's really no way around it. Setting realistic goals when you're traveling can feel similar to shooting at a constantly-moving target. But, with time and practice, you'll eventually become a pro at sticking to your fitness goals on the road.

To do this, you'll first have to carefully consider the various constraints that come with travel, like the ones we mentioned above. This is where short, gymless bodyweight workouts come in handy. Your fitness goals may need to become a little bit more lax while you're traveling in order to accommodate the changing setting. Additionally, adaptability is key, so you'll want to opt for exercises that can be performed in diverse or changing settings. In the next few sections, we'll cover some options to achieve this.

Designing Flexible Workout Plans for Travel

First, let's talk about packing for success. In previous chapters, you learned a bit about all of the different apps and trackers that the digital age can offer fitness enthusiasts. All of these options—from scheduling to workout ideas—are doubly useful while you're on the road.

That being said, only doing bodyweight exercises can sometimes feel a little bland and boring. Bodyweight exercising can feel like the only real option while traveling, and while it works just as well as any other exercise, longer trips may require a little extra motivation in the form of equipment. With limited space and weight allotments for flights, travelers should prioritize options that are small, lightweight, and easily packed. Believe it or not, several choices fit this description, such as:

- resistance bands

- jump rope

- swimwear

- wearable weights

- core sliders

To get the most metaphorical bang for your buck, it's also worth checking out your local amenities. Most hotels have pools, outdoor spaces, and small gyms with all the equipment you need—if you know that this will be the case for your next trip, you may even consider skipping portable workout equipment altogether.

Integrating Fitness Into Travel Itineraries

Unfortunately, you won't always have time during the workday to get in some extra movement. When you do, you can consult the methods we talked about in Chapter 6 for inspiration. The biggest issues you'll face—like soreness, stiffness, and sustained sitting—arise while you're actually in transit. For now, we'll talk about some of the things you can do to get your blood pumping when you have minimal space.

Staying Active During Transit

It may seem like a stretch, but you can actually get in some movement while in transit. Whether you're flying, driving, or riding in passenger transit, there are always things you can do to get your blood pumping, even if it's not a full workout. By now, you already know: Fitness is a lifestyle choice, not a time or place!

More space is ideal, of course, but even the most packed flight still offers some wiggle room for exercises like these:

- Knee circles. When you're in a sitting position, like on a plane or in a train car, this is a great mini-workout. First, make sure you're sitting up straight, with your head and chest held up. Press your palms down on the seat on either side of you. One leg at a time, slowly lift your knee and rotate it in a circular motion, careful not to let the ball of your foot hit the ground. After a couple of reps, repeat with the other leg.

- Stand-on-fists. If your wrists are injured or sensitive, you may want to skip this exercise. For this exercise, you'll start in the same way that you started your knee circles. This time, you'll want to make your hands into fists rather than putting your weight on your open palms. Slowly, shift your weight onto your fists until most of your weight is carried by them. If you can, raise yourself off the seat just a little bit. Hold this for a few seconds, then lower yourself back onto the seat and slowly shift your weight back onto your bum.

- Flexed eagle. The seated version of this yoga pose will help you flex your arms and stretch out your back at the same time. Sitting normally, reach both of your arms out in front of you and then cross your left elbow over the upper portion of your right arm. From here, bring both arms into a vertical position and clasp your palms together. Flex and sustain the pose for a few minutes, then repeat with the other side.

Whether stationary or in transit, business people are often fatigued by the end of the workday. Sometimes, this can seep into your fitness routines and manifest in some nasty side effects. In the next chapter, we'll explore fatigue, where it comes from, and what you can do to counteract it in the long run—no pun intended.

Chapter 9:

From Fatigued to Energized—Overcoming Mental and Physical Fatigue

According to a 2020 poll from the National Sleep Foundation, Americans feel sleepy during the day a whopping three days out of the week (Langer Research Associates, 2020). While the poll didn't assess the sleep or health habits of all Americans, it's safe to say that a lot of people feel consistently fatigued throughout the week. The danger for those in the business world is greater than the average person's, making fatigue during the day an all too common experience that inhibits productivity, worsens mood, and wrecks your physical health.

Understanding Fatigue in the Professional World

In recent years, society has become increasingly aware of the effects of burnout and burnout-like conditions. Professionals, and especially business owners, probably know this feeling well. Over time, burnout and general fatigue can take a massive toll on your mental health, physical well-being, and professional productivity.

For those who are seeking to maintain fitness routines, this can be a very dangerous place to land—before you know it, something that felt like a simple off-day turns into a persisting feeling of fatigue and a lack of motivation. As such, it's crucial to know what the beginnings of persistent fatigue might feel like, even if they're only small symptoms. Anxiety over looming work tasks, increasing physical tiredness, wandering attention, and difficulty focusing can all turn into something long-lasting, inevitably affecting your health outcomes. Sometimes, feelings as innocuous as frustration can be indicators of something bigger if occurring repeatedly.

One of the best things you can do to prevent persistent fatigue is to equip yourself with knowledge about where it comes from, particularly at work. Some of the most common sources of mental fatigue include:

- lifestyle choices

- medical issues and illnesses

- workplace stress

Ultimately, the best way to minimize the fatigue you feel at work is to treat the root of the issue. When the source is gone, there's a far smaller chance that the fatigue will leach into your fitness routines.

The Vicious Cycle of Fatigue and Inactivity

Like many aspects of your physical health, fatigue is often cyclical. It usually starts with prolonged periods of inactivity or sedentary behavior, leading to muscle weakness, decreased cardiovascular fitness, and a decline in overall energy levels. As physical activity decreases, the body's metabolism slows down, which in turn can contribute to weight gain and decreased motivation for exercise. This decline in physical health can also impact your mental well-being, leading to feelings of lethargy, low moods, and increased stress levels. Fatigue sets in, making it more challenging to engage in regular physical activity. The cycle perpetuates as fatigue and inactivity reinforce each other, creating a loop that hinders overall wellness.

This terrible and exhausting cycle inevitably seeps back into your professional life, making work feel harder and working out feel nearly impossible. Ironically, the best way to break the loop is by making yourself temporarily more tired through exercise during the day.

Strategies to Overcome Fatigue Through Exercise

While you might not feel like doing anything when you're fatigued, mindful and intentional workouts can help you regain some of your energy. Once you get over the initial hump of inertia, you'll probably end up feeling far better than you otherwise would. This isn't just a theory, either: Science has long proven that exercise can actually boost your overall energy levels—provided that you exercise effectively.

In one finding, Doctors Tina Golen and Hope Ricciotti explain that exercising when you feel fatigued changes your body chemistry on a cellular level. There are basically three ways this happens. First, exertion—like that which occurs during high-intensity workouts—prompts your body's cells to produce more mitochondria. Mitochondria are crucial in turning the glucose you consume into usable energy for your body's cells, so more mitochondrial work effectively allows more physical work to be done. In other words, consistent exercise means that your cells are more readily available to give your muscles the energy they need to move. Additionally, the same process of exertion increases the oxygen levels in your blood, which plays a key role in the effectiveness of cell function. In your brain, exercise also releases certain hormones like dopamine, which influences your emotions and further facilitates your physiology (Golen & Ricciotti, 2021).

Long story short, exercise of all kinds has the potential to give you energy and get you over the wall of fatigue you might be feeling. That said, some exercises are just immediate energy-boosters, such as:

- jogging

- swimming

- walking outside

- stretching and yoga

In these cases, your setting and method of performance can also play a role in the effectiveness of exercising. Instead of dragging yourself out of your office chair for a boring jog, try doing your best Bruce Lee kicks. The next time you suspect that fatigue is creeping into your day, bust out the most ridiculous dance move you can muster—you'll be moving your body and probably having fun in the process.

Creating an Energizing Workout Environment

Sometimes, your surroundings are the best place to start when you feel fatigued. If going for a five-mile run doesn't sound very appealing, try at least prepping your space for your next workout. This is a great starting point for people who prefer to work out from home or for frequent travelers who start feeling fatigued while on the road. To start, consider some of the following:

- Tidy and clean your space to encourage yourself to move around.

- Take a look at the floors, and consider getting workout mats that you can lay down to soften the impact of hard flooring.

- Consider new storage options, particularly ones that place your workout equipment in plain view—while still being tidy.

- Crack open a window to let natural light in.

Lifestyle Adjustments to Enhance Energy

As you might imagine, feeling consistently fatigued also has ties to other areas of your health and well-being. For one, feeling sleepy during the day inevitably comes back to your sleep habits at night, including sleep quality, duration, and potential interruptions.

Improving Sleep Quality

It might sound like a lazy choice, but sleep can be the key to overcoming bouts of fatigue. For those who are just starting to dive into daily workouts—or workouts of any kind, for that matter—this is nothing to be ashamed of. Contrary to many self-imposed ideas about laziness and shortcuts, ensuring a full night's rest with a good quality of sleep is a great way to make sure you stay awake during the day. The idea of sleep as a self-care activity is relatively new, but it's given rise to a new scientific and medical niche that's commonly referred to as sleep hygiene.

Sleep hygiene takes the same approach to sleep as we do with normal bodily hygiene, like showering and brushing our teeth. For busy professionals, many of whom often pride themselves on how little sleep they get, this may be a tough pill to swallow. However, studies have shown that taking proper care of your sleep habits can improve productivity, cognitive function, and general physical health. Subsequently, it's in your best interests to understand how to improve your sleep! In this setting, there are a couple of science-backed steps you can take to improve your sleep (*Sleep Hygiene Tips*, 2022), such as:

- maintaining a consistent sleep schedule wake-up times and sleep times

- consistently sleeping in dark, quiet spaces

- ditching electronics at least an hour—preferably more—before bed

- avoiding large meals, caffeine, alcohol, and other substances before sleep

- exercising throughout the day

If you're really feeling tired during the day, naps aren't strictly outlawed when it comes to good sleep hygiene. That being said, most sources recommend that naps stay under 30 minutes in length and that you only nap in the early afternoons (Suni, 2020).

As terrible as it is, fatigue is something that will always pose a potential risk along your fitness journey. Like busy schedules and limited resources, fatigue is just something that you'll have to learn to live with. The alternative—living a sedentary lifestyle, worsening your mood and productivity, and leaving yourself open to health-related illnesses and conditions—is far worse. In the next chapter, we'll talk about how to change your mindset about fitness in the long run, particularly when the going gets rough.

Chapter 10

Building a Fitness Mindset in a Busy World

It may be cliche to point out, but our collective mindset about fitness and health is typically a very privileged one. It's not until we encounter serious sickness, illnesses, or other big life events that we stop and reconsider our conceptions—and misconceptions.

This was the case for one busy professional and single mom, Julie. It wasn't until her daughter, Elena, was diagnosed at an early age with neuroblastoma, which in turn compressed Elena's spine and paralyzed her from the waist down. According to one account of Julie's story:

> [Julie, Elena's mother] sought out therapy; she also began running to manage her extreme depression. Those interventions helped, but Julie's challenges soon became physical, as well; As Elena grew, it became more difficult for Julie to her pick up and carry her.

As the situation for this mother and daughter worsened, one of Julie's trainers suggested Julie try Olympic weightlifting. Intimidated but inspired, she learned the basics from her trainer... Fast-forward, Elena's now 130 lbs and... she lifts her daughter easily. Now, both Julie and Elena are happy and healthy, in part due to their mindset about their own health. Despite being paralyzed from the waist down, Elena trains with her mom every day. For them, fitness is a bonding exercise that strengthens their physical and mental health, brings them closer together, and reminds them of how far they've come: "Julie's own physical strength—she now trains 2 hours a day, 7 days a week—and her hard-won insights as the parent of a disabled child have given her emotional resilience and perspective" (Patton, n.d.).

Cultivating the Right Mindset for Fitness

For many of us, we may never reach Julie and Elena's drive for fitness. However, we can still look at their story and follow their amazing example. Ultimately, fitness isn't just a means to an end; it's just as much about the journey as it is about the result.

Understanding the Psychology of Fitness

At this point, you've—hopefully—adopted the idea that fitness is a lifestyle choice, not a one-time activity committed only in certain settings. Saying this is easy, and even proving this scientifically is easy—changing your mindset, on the other hand, isn't always the easiest task. As you grow and learn on your fitness journey, your mindset about fitness itself will also grow and change. This is a beautiful process, but we often encounter moments in which our definitions of fitness and health can't change fast enough.

Using mindfulness, there are ways that you can slowly adapt your understanding of fitness into one that's more accurate— and beneficial to you.

It won't always be easy, but keep an eye out for moments like these:

- Opportunities to revise your self-talk: Oftentimes, we think of our own bodies as doing either a *good* or bad job. While congratulating and encouraging yourself is a great step toward changing the narrative around fitness, thinking in black-and-white terms isn't always the best way forward. Instead, try to cultivate a growth mindset in which you recognize that improvement is always possible—even when you're struggling.

- Chances for redefinition: Even when we rationally know that exercise isn't limited to a certain time or place, we can still catch ourselves thinking in outdated terms. When this happens, it's worth reminding ourselves that exercise is just moving our body.

- Memories and present-moment feelings: When you're struggling, try to think about a time when exercising made you feel good, either mentally or physically. Chances are, there are several instances you might think of, like playing volleyball with friends or kayaking down a beautiful river. These memories will help you think more holistically about your fitness experience.

- Keeping your eye on the prize: Again, fitness isn't just a means to an end. That being said, the *end* is still an important aspect of your motivations. In times of struggle or fatigue, consider why you started your fitness journey in the first place.

Over time, you'll find that doing fitness activities you enjoy actually stops being a chore. With time, mindfulness, and consistency, you may start looking forward to your daily workouts as a reprieve from the worries of the world. In essence, fitness is the ultimate mechanism of self-care you can pursue, ensuring your health for now and for the future.

Harnessing the Power of Habits and Routines

The initial step toward establishing a sustainable routine involves turning your health into a habit. First, let's make a distinction between the two; simply put, a routine is something that you do periodically. A habit, on the other hand, is an automated, subconscious aspect of daily life, such as basic hygiene or blinking. You don't actively think about flipping the light switch when you walk into a dark room; you just do it out of habit. Ingrained routines, like brushing your teeth or flipping a light switch, seamlessly integrate into your everyday life without requiring extra effort. As a result, it's difficult to ditch habits altogether. Breaking them requires usually more effort than it took to form them in the first place. When it comes to fitness, you can use this information to your advantage.

For busy professionals who want to make fitness into a habit, the journey from consciously-performed routine to habit can pose a bit of a tricky challenge. At first, you'll need to put in more effort to perform the actions you want to turn into habits. One approach you could take involves focusing on small adjustments, like putting on your running shoes after breakfast or charging your Bluetooth headphones before you go to bed. You can't make *being fit* into a habit all at once, but you can certainly start preparing yourself for success with small pieces of fitness that you automate over time.

Another approach to habit formation suggests making the act of working out as effortless as possible while still maintaining its health benefits and structure. Considering your physical and mental environment before, during, and after your daily workout is crucial. According to James Clear, author of *Atomic Habits*, elements like time, location, preceding events, and emotional state play pivotal roles in building effective habits:

1. Time and preceding events: Time is easily measurable, which makes it a great way to build habits. Integrating new habits becomes easier when you align them with existing routines, making them a part of your habitual repertoire, so to speak. This is the concept of preceding events, and it's very useful for building new habits. In practice, it goes something like this: You have two habits that you do every day, like turning on the coffee pot and brushing your teeth. In between these two habits, there's a window of time that you could use to your advantage, perhaps by doing some lunges or a couple of burpees. You may hear some sources call this habit-stacking.

2. Location: Choosing diverse settings for activities can sometimes help form associations, making you more inclined to stay on track. The key here is to choose somewhere you don't normally go or somewhere less common and start associating it with working out. This could be a traditional gym, or it could be a trail near your home. Fitness shouldn't generally be isolated to particular places and times, but in this instance, picking a consistent location is key to getting the ball rolling.

3. Emotional state: I don't know about you, but I was actually taught about the dangers of emotional state in driver's ed. Getting behind the wheel when you're absolutely distraught can be a dangerous choice. While my driving instructor meant this in a literal sense, the

idea also has metaphorical meaning—when you're dealing with tough emotions, trying to make the right choice feels harder. Inversely, you can also use your emotional state to prompt you to take steps toward your fitness goals. Let me explain what I mean: If you've just left a stressful meeting at work, you might not be consciously aware of your stress levels. After acknowledging that you're feeling stressed, you can try to minimize this problem by doing something calming like taking a walk, doing yoga, or any of the stress-busting exercises we discussed in Chapter 3.

Using these techniques, you can slowly start turning small fitness-related tasks into habits you automatically do, prompting you to engage in fitness activities and preparing you for success.

Chapter 11:

Workout Plans for All Occasions

If you do a quick Google search, you'll find there are countless resources to pick from when it comes to hashing out a specific workout routine. When you add up these myriad online sources with your in-person options, like gyms and classes, you'll find that the possibilities are quite endless. In fact, workout plans make up a huge sector of an additionally booming health and fitness niche—according to industry research company IBISWorld, U.S. health and fitness businesses alone have seen a 2.3% increase from 2022–2023 (*Industry Market Research*, 2023).

That may not sound like a lot at first, but let's do some quick math. There's an estimated total of 113,326 U.S.-based fitness companies in existence today. For reference, that's more than double all of the McDonald's, Starbucks, Burger King, Pizza Hut, and Subway locations *combined* (*Number of Burger King Locations*, 2024; *Number of Pizza Hut Locations*, 2024; *Number of Starbucks locations*, 2024). For even more reference, there are only about 6,146 active hospitals in the US (*105 Hospital Statistics*, 2023). Given the U.S.'s total current population as of writing—a little over 336 million people—that means there's 1 fitness company for every 2,965 people. Additionally, these numbers don't take multinational businesses into account. In other words, there's no lack of fitness opinions out there. To complicate matters even more, there's no surefire way to know which opinions will provide safe and effective workout options for you.

All of this can be quite overwhelming to consider, especially if you're just starting to workout consistently for the first time. Unfortunately, this wealth of information may start to contribute to a sense of disenfranchisement, ultimately dissuading you from trying out new workout routines.

Luckily, you've already tackled the hardest part of this process: getting started! Just by thinking about the next steps in your fitness journey, you've already started to break down the barriers that stop you from adopting a new workout routine. To stave off the overwhelm and keep you motivated, let's streamline all of this information down to the most common and most effective workout routines out there. In addition to some basic templates, we'll implement some of the scheduling techniques we've talked about in the past 10 chapters. Location by location, let's take a look at a basic workout structure and ways that you might spice it up.

The Basic Routine

Before we start looking at specific locations, let's take a look at a basic workout structure that you can use in all situations. While spontaneity can boost your sense of motivation, having a basic routine or rhythm in your back pocket can make working out feel like far less of a chore. For each of the situations we'll be covering here, we'll outline several exercises that are adaptable for both time-based HIIT routines and repetition-based circuits.

To start, a basic HIIT or circuit structure might look something like this:

Warm-up	Exercise 1	Exercise 2	Exercise 3	Exercise 4	Cooldown
5 minutes	5 minutes	5 minutes	5 minutes	5 minutes	5 minutes

This example outlines a 30-minute workout, but as we've said in the previous chapters, HIIT is highly adaptable, allowing you to create shorter routines depending on the situation. Additionally, it's a good idea to incorporate brief rest times—anywhere from 30 seconds to 1 minute—after each of your main exercises.

Alternatively, repetition-based circuit routines may look more like this:

Warm-up	Exercise 1	Exercise 2	Exercise 3	Exercise 4	Cooldown
5 minutes	10 reps, 2 sets	10 reps, 2 sets	10 reps, 2 sets	10 reps, 2 sets	5 minutes

As with the HIIT outline, it's worth mentioning that the number of core exercises, repetitions, and sets you choose to include can be adapted to fit your situation. Here, rest times may be incorporated between sets or between exercises.

Exercise Options for Every Scenario

Before we dive in, there are two things we should take note of with regard to exercises. Firstly, this is by no means a comprehensive list! Part of long-term fitness and motivation is seeking out new knowledge as you progress. Rather, this list is a jumping-off point for those who want to simplify their routines.

Secondly, it's crucial that you consult your doctor before adopting any new exercises or workout routines. This is even more pertinent for those who have preexisting health conditions or chronic illnesses. More often than not, your doctor will probably have some ideas about how to make exercises and workouts more accessible to your level, which will boost the results you see in the long run.

For our purposes, we'll also make distinctions between warm-up exercises, cool-down exercises, and main exercises, as these will vary slightly in intensity. In other words, our goal here is to provide you with some basic exercises that will allow you to *plug-and-chug*, so to speak, with location-specific routines. Additionally, while you might be familiar with a number of these exercises, others might be new to you. With this in mind, let's explore your exercise choices and how to perform each one correctly.

Warm-ups

- **Ankle rotations:** This straightforward exercise can be performed either seated on a chair or standing. Lift one foot off the ground, ensuring a 90° bend at the knee if sitting, or shift your weight to one leg if standing. Begin the exercise by smoothly rotating your ankle clockwise, imagining a circle traced by your big toe. Focus on engaging the full range of motion from the ankle joint. After several rotations, switch to counterclockwise movements. Repeat the entire process for the other ankle. It's crucial to maintain controlled and deliberate motions, avoiding any abrupt or forceful movements.

Ankle rotations contribute to improved flexibility and joint mobility and can be seamlessly integrated into warm-up routines to prevent stiffness and discomfort. However, individuals with existing ankle issues should consult healthcare professionals or physical therapists before incorporating this exercise.

- **Arm circles:** For this, we're going to take everything we just described for ankle rotations and apply it to your arms. To start, stand with your feet shoulder-width apart and extend your arms out to the sides at shoulder height, forming a T-shape with your body. Engage your core muscles for stability and initiate small clockwise circular motions from the shoulder joint, gradually increasing the diameter as your shoulders loosen up. After a period, switch to counterclockwise circles. Strive for a full range of motion, keeping your shoulders relaxed. You can customize the size of the circles and vary the palm direction for an added challenge. Arm circles are an effective addition to warm-up routines, preparing the shoulders for more intense physical activities, improving flexibility, and reducing the risk of injury.

- **Jumping jacks:** You probably had to do jumping jacks when you were in grade school physical education classes, but a quick refresher may still be beneficial. Start in a standing position with feet together and arms relaxed at your sides, maintaining good posture. As you jump, simultaneously spread your legs apart and raise your arms above your head to form an "X" shape. Land softly on the balls of your feet with a slight bend in your knees, bringing your arms back down to your sides. It's crucial to focus on the quality of the movement, emphasizing fluidity over speed and engaging your core throughout.

- **Wall push-ups:** You've likely done push-ups, but wall push-ups provide an easier and more accessible workout. This can either be a warmup or a starter exercise if you're not comfortable doing full sets of push-ups yet. To start, stand at an arm's length away from a wall with your feet shoulder-width apart. Place your hands on the wall at shoulder height, slightly wider than shoulder width. Engage your core to maintain a straight line from head to heels. Inhale as you bend your elbows, lowering your chest toward the wall, and exhale as you push away, straightening your arms back to the starting position. Focus on controlled movements and proper hand placement. Gradually adjust the difficulty by varying the distance between you and the wall. Wall push-ups work your chest muscles, shoulders, and triceps.

- **High knees:** High knees are kind of like jogging in place, but the exercise emphasizes height rather than the speed of your stride. This also engages your legs, core, and hip flexors, making it a great way to kickstart more intense workouts. Start by standing tall with feet hip-width apart, ensuring proper posture. Engage your core muscles for stability and lift one knee toward your chest, alternating with a running or marching motion. Coordinate the movement by swinging your arms in tandem with your legs, maintaining a brisk pace to elevate your heart rate. Land softly on the balls of your feet with each descent, and strive for a full range of motion by lifting your knees as high as comfortable.

- **Seat squeezes:** Seat squeezes, also known as glute squeezes, are a simple yet effective exercise to activate and strengthen the muscles in your buttocks. To perform seat squeezes, start by sitting comfortably on a chair with your feet flat on the floor, shoulder-width apart. Engage your core muscles to maintain proper posture. Slowly squeeze your buttocks together, holding the contraction for a few seconds, and then release. Focus on isolating the glute muscles and avoid overarching your lower back. Seat squeezes can be done discreetly throughout the day, making them an excellent option for toning the glutes and improving overall lower body strength, especially for those with a sedentary lifestyle or those looking for a convenient seated exercise.

- **Deep breathing:** Deep breathing, sometimes also referred to as diaphragmatic or abdominal breathing, is a simple and effective technique to promote relaxation and reduce stress. To practice deep breathing, find a comfortable seated or lying position. Place one hand on your chest and the other on your abdomen. Inhale deeply through your nose, allowing your diaphragm to expand and your abdomen to rise. Exhale slowly and completely through your mouth, feeling your abdomen fall. Focus on breathing deeply into your lower lungs, allowing your chest to remain relatively still. Repeat this process for several breaths, aiming for a slow and controlled rhythm.

- **Torso twists:** Torso twists enhance spinal mobility and engage the core muscles, which may be ideal for more rigorous workouts. Start by sitting or standing with a straight spine. Place your hands on your hips or clasp them together in front of you. Slowly rotate your upper body to one side, keeping your hips facing forward. Allow your gaze to follow the movement, and feel the stretch across your midsection. Hold the position for a few seconds, then return to the center. Repeat the twist to the opposite side. Maintain a controlled and gentle pace throughout the exercise, avoiding any jerky movements.

- **Shoulder blade squeezes:** Shoulder blade squeezes are a simple exercise to improve posture and strengthen the muscles between your shoulder blades. Begin by sitting or standing with a straight spine. Relax your shoulders and bring them down, away from your ears. Slowly squeeze your shoulder blades together as if you are trying to hold a small object between them. Hold the squeeze for a few seconds, feeling the contraction in your upper back, and then release. Shoulder blade squeezes can be done discreetly throughout the day to counteract the effects of slouching and promote better shoulder alignment.

Main Exercises

- **Chair squats:** Chair squats are a straightforward and effective exercise that targets the muscles in your lower body, particularly the quadriceps, hamstrings, and glutes. To perform chair squats, start by standing in front of a sturdy chair with your feet shoulder-width apart. Engage your core for stability. Lower your body by bending at your hips and knees as if you were sitting back in the chair. Keep your chest lifted and ensure your knees stay in line with your toes. Hover just above the chair without fully sitting down, then press through your heels to return to the starting position.

- **Seated leg raises:** Seated leg raises are a targeted exercise to strengthen the muscles in your lower abdominal area and thighs. To perform seated leg raises, start by sitting on a sturdy chair with your back straight and feet flat on the floor. Hold onto the sides of the chair for stability. Lift one leg straight out in front of you, keeping it parallel to the ground. Hold for a moment, engaging your core muscles, and then slowly lower the leg back down without letting it touch the floor. Repeat the movement on the other leg.

- **Wall sits:** Wall sits are an effective lower body exercise that targets the quadriceps, hamstrings, and glutes. To perform wall sits, find a clear wall and stand with your back against it. Slowly slide down the wall, bending your knees until they are at a 90° angle, resembling a seated position. Ensure your knees are directly above your ankles and your back is flat against the wall. Hold this seated position for as long as you can, aiming for at least 30 seconds to a minute. Focus on maintaining good posture with your core engaged. As you build strength, you can gradually increase the duration of the wall sit.

- **Calf raises:** Calf raises are a simple yet effective exercise that targets the muscles in your calves. To perform calf raises, start by standing with your feet hip-width apart on a flat surface. Keep your core engaged for stability. Slowly rise up onto the balls of your feet by lifting your heels off the ground as high as you can. Hold the raised position for a moment, feeling the contraction in your calf muscles, and then lower your heels back down below the level of the platform. To increase the challenge, you can perform calf raises on an elevated surface.

- **Desk–chair dips:** Dips are a straightforward and effective exercise that targets the muscles in your triceps and shoulders. To perform desk–chair dips, begin by sitting on the edge of a sturdy chair or desk with your hands gripping the front edge and fingers facing forward. Slide your hips forward, lowering your body off the chair while keeping your feet flat on the floor and knees bent at a 90° angle. Lower your body until your elbows are bent at about a 90° angle, then push through your palms to lift your body back up to the starting position.

- **Abdominal contractions:** Sitting abdominal contractions are a subtle yet effective exercise to engage and strengthen your core muscles. Begin by sitting comfortably on a chair with your back straight and feet flat on the floor. Place your hands on your thighs for support. Inhale deeply, engaging your abdominal muscles by pulling your belly button toward your spine. Hold this contraction for a few seconds, feeling the tension in your core, and then exhale as you release.

The key is to focus on the controlled engagement of your abdominal muscles without involving other muscle groups.

- **Overhead press:** Start by standing with your feet shoulder-width apart. Hold a dumbbell in each hand, positioning them at shoulder height with your palms facing forward. Engage your core for stability and ensure a neutral spine. Inhale, then exhale as you press the dumbbells overhead by fully extending your arms. Keep your wrists aligned with your elbows throughout the movement. Pause briefly at the top, feeling the contraction in your shoulders, and then lower the dumbbells back to shoulder height. Overhead presses effectively target the deltoid muscles in your shoulders and also engage your triceps. Ensure proper form to avoid unnecessary strain, and gradually increase the weight as your strength improves.

- **Lateral raises:** To perform lat raises, start by standing with your feet hip-width apart, holding a dumbbell in each hand hanging by each side of your body, with your palms facing your body. Maintain a slight bend in your elbows throughout the exercise. Engage your core for stability and lift the dumbbells out to the sides until your arms are parallel to the floor. Focus on using your shoulder muscles to lift the weights, avoiding excessive swinging or momentum. Hold the raised position for a moment to maximize the contraction in your lateral deltoids, then lower the dumbbells back down with control. Lateral raises effectively target the lateral— outer—part of your shoulders, contributing to a well-rounded shoulder development.

- **Weighted lunges:** Weighted lunges are an effective lower body exercise that adds resistance to target the muscles in your legs and glutes. To start, hold a dumbbell in each hand, positioning them at your sides with your palms facing inward. Stand with your feet together. Take a step forward with one foot, ensuring your knee is directly above your ankle, forming a 90° angle. Lower your body by bending both knees, keeping your back straight and chest lifted. Push through your front heel to return to the starting position. Repeat with the other leg for a complete repetition. Weighted lunges provide an excellent way to challenge and strengthen your quadriceps, hamstrings, and glutes.

- **Decline push-ups:** To perform decline push-ups, position yourself in a push-up stance with your hands on the floor and your feet elevated on a sturdy surface, such as a bench or step, creating a decline angle. Ensure your hands are slightly wider than shoulder-width apart. Engage your core, keeping your body in a straight line from head to heels. Lower your chest toward the floor by bending your elbows, then push back up to the starting position. The decline angle intensifies the resistance on your chest, shoulders, and triceps, offering a more challenging variation of the traditional push-up.

- **Pistol squats:** Pistol squats, also known as single-leg squats, are a challenging and effective exercise that targets your quadriceps, hamstrings, and glutes. Begin by standing on one leg with your foot firmly planted on the ground. Extend the opposite leg straight in front of you, keeping it parallel to the ground. Lower your body into a squat position by bending your standing knee, ensuring it tracks over your toes. Keep your back straight, your chest lifted, and your arms extended for balance. Aim to lower your body until your thigh is parallel to the ground or as far as your mobility allows. Press through your heel to return to the starting position. Pistol squats require strength, balance, and flexibility, so it's essential to start with a partial range of motion and gradually progress as your strength improves.

- **Plank leg lift:** Plank leg lifts are a dynamic variation of the traditional plank exercise, focusing on engaging the core and targeting the muscles in your lower body. Start in a plank position with your hands directly under your shoulders and your body forming a straight line from head to heels. Lift one leg off the ground, extending it straight back while keeping your hips level. Hold the leg at the highest point for a moment, engaging your glutes and maintaining stability through your core. Lower the leg back down and switch to the other leg. Ensure your hips stay parallel to the ground throughout the exercise to maximize effectiveness.

- **Weighted Russian twists:** Weighted Russian twists are a challenging exercise that engages the core, especially the obliques. Begin by sitting on the floor with your knees bent and your feet flat on the ground. Hold a weight or a medicine ball with both hands, extending your arms in front of you. Lean back slightly to engage your core muscles. Lift your feet off the ground, balancing on your sit bones. Twist your torso to one side, bringing the weight or medicine ball beside your hip. Return to the center and then twist to the other side. Weighted Russian twists effectively target the muscles along your sides, contributing to improved core strength and stability. Adjust the weight according to your fitness level, gradually increasing it as your strength progresses.

- **Mountain climbers:** Mountain climbers are a dynamic and full-body exercise that targets the core, shoulders, and legs. Start in a plank position with your hands directly under your shoulders, forming a straight line from head to heels. Engage your core and bring one knee toward your chest, then quickly switch and bring the other knee in while extending the first leg back. Continue alternating your legs in a running motion, keeping your hips level and your core tight. Focus on maintaining proper form and a consistent rhythm to maximize the effectiveness of this dynamic exercise.

- **Pull-ups:** Pull-ups are a potent upper body exercise that primarily targets the muscles in your back, including the latissimus dorsi. Find a sturdy horizontal bar, such as a pull-up bar, and grip it with your palms facing away from you, slightly wider than shoulder-width apart. Hang from the bar with your arms fully extended. Engage your core and, using the strength of your back and arms, pull your body upward until your chin clears the bar. Lower yourself back down with control, fully extending your arms. If pull-ups are challenging initially, consider using assistance from a pull-up band or a pull-up machine.

- **Burpees:** Burpees are a full-body, high-intensity exercise that combines strength training and cardio. Start by standing with your feet shoulder-width apart. Drop into a squat position, placing your hands on the ground. Jump your feet back, landing in a plank position. Perform a push-up, then jump your feet back toward your hands. Explosively jump up from the squat position, reaching your arms overhead. Land softly and immediately go into the next repetition.

Cooldowns

- **Step-ups:** Step-ups are a straightforward yet effective cool-down exercise that targets the muscles in your legs and glutes. Begin by standing in front of a sturdy bench or step. Place one foot on the bench, ensuring your entire foot is secure on the surface. Press through the heel of the elevated foot, engage your core, and lift your body onto the bench. Straighten your hip and knee on the elevated leg before bringing the opposite leg up to meet it. Step back down with the same leading leg, followed by the other.

- **Forward folds:** A forward fold, also known as Uttanasana in yoga, is a calming and rejuvenating stretch that targets the hamstrings and lower back. Start by standing with your feet hip-width apart and your knees slightly bent. Inhale deeply, lengthening your spine, and as you exhale, hinge your hips to fold forward. Allow your upper body to hang over your legs, and let your head and neck relax. You can bend your knees as much as needed, especially if you're a beginner or have tight hamstrings. Hold onto your shins, ankles, or the floor, depending on your flexibility. Feel the stretch along the back of your legs and aim to bring your chest closer to your thighs with each breath. Hold the position for 30 seconds to a minute, then slowly rise back up to a standing position.

- **Quad stretches:** Performing a quad stretch is beneficial for flexibility and can help alleviate tightness in the quadriceps. Begin by standing on one leg with your feet hip-width apart. If needed, use a sturdy object like a chair or wall for balance. Bend your other knee, bringing the heel toward your buttocks, and grab your ankle with the hand on the same side. Gently pull your ankle toward your buttocks while keeping your knees close together. Ensure that your standing knee is pointing straight ahead and your thighs are parallel. Switch to the other leg and repeat.

- **Chest openers:** Chest openers are an excellent stretch to release tension in the chest, shoulders, and upper back. Begin by standing or sitting with a straight spine. Clasp your hands together behind your back, straightening your arms. If clasping your hands isn't accessible, you can use a towel or a yoga strap to bridge the gap between your hands. Lift your arms slightly and open your chest by squeezing your shoulder blades together. Allow your gaze to lift, opening the front of your neck. Chest openers are beneficial for counteracting the effects of prolonged sitting, promoting better posture, and enhancing overall upper body flexibility. Incorporate them into your stretching routine or perform them periodically throughout the day to relieve tension in the chest and improve the range of motion in the shoulders.

- **Child's pose:** Child's Pose, or Balasana in yoga, is a restorative and relaxing stretch that targets the back, hips, and thighs. Begin by kneeling on the mat with your big toes touching and knees spread apart. Sit back on your heels and exhale as you lower your torso between your thighs. Extend your arms forward on the mat with your palms down, allowing your forehead to rest on the floor. Keep your arms active, pressing into the mat, and lengthen through your spine. Feel the gentle stretch along your back and hips.

Home Workout Routine

When working out at home, you should consider a few basic things before you start your routine. For one, you should always make sure that your space is clear of obstacles, objects, or falling hazards, and it might be a good idea to tidy up before your workout. It's also a great idea to designate a particular workout area in your home—like the living room—so that you can start establishing an association between your space and your workouts. This will ultimately help you in forming the long-term habits that we talked about in the last chapter.

With regard to the content of your home workouts, you should pay attention to a couple of things. Limited space to move and limited time are certainly big factors, but the biggest thing you should focus on is equipment—or the lack thereof. If you have at-home workout equipment like a treadmill or a squat rack, now is definitely the time to bust them out! However, most people don't have weights or machines at home. If you're in this boat, lack of equipment isn't a reason to skimp on your workout. Rather, your home workout should revolve primarily around bodyweight exercises.

Once you've designated a workout space, it's time to get to work! If you're doing a time-based HIIT workout, set your timer and get started on a basic routine like this:

- **warm-up—1 minute per exercise, 5 minutes total:**

    - jumping jacks

    - high knees

    - butt kicks

    - arm circles

    - bodyweight squats

- **five main cycles—1 minute per exercise, 5 minutes per cycle:**

    - pistol squats

    - push-ups

    - mountain climbers

    - burpees

    - plank—30 seconds

    - 30-second rest

- **cooldown—1 minute per exercise, 5 minutes total:**

    ○ slow jogging in place

    ○ step-ups

    ○ seated hamstring stretch

    ○ chest opener stretch

    ○ child's pose

As you can see, the transition between exercises is rapid, and each exercise is limited to one minute only. Knowing this, it may be helpful for you to have a clock or a timer in your line of sight so that you can effectively stick to the one-minute limit. Personally, I like to set my phone down on the floor next to where I'm working out so that I can periodically check my progress. You may also want to lower the number of cycles you perform, depending on your scheduling needs. If you'd rather count your repetitions of each exercise—given that you're doing exercises with repetitions—instead of timing yourself, this is also a viable option.

Office Workout

When you're at the office, you probably won't have as much room to work out as you would at home. You may be confined to your desk area or working out in a smaller break area. Ideally, parking lots or garages will provide more room to move, so outdoor spaces are preferable when possible. However, don't let your space dictate your fitness! If you're stuck at your desk for prolonged stretches of time, you'll want to squeeze in a workout that's space-efficient, quiet, and nondisruptive to coworkers or colleagues around you. To get you thinking, here's a basic template for a quick 20-minute workout:

- **warm-up—1 minute per exercise, 5 minutes total:**

  - ankle circles

  - torso twists

  - wall push-ups

  - arm circles

  - deep breathing

- **two main cycles—1 minute per exercise, 5 minutes per cycle:**

  - desk–chair dips

  - seated leg raises

  - chair squats

  - wall sits

  - lunges

- **cooldown—about 1 minute per exercise, 5 minutes total:**

  - quad stretches

  - standing forward fold

- chest opener stretch

- neck and shoulder stretching

Outdoor Workout

Outdoor workouts are some of the most fun and effective workouts you can do. If you can get out into nature—like on a trail or at a park—all the better! Outdoor workouts give you a much wider variety of activities to choose from, many of which you wouldn't find in a home workout or a gym routine. Even if you don't have access to equipment, you can still find things like park benches, playgrounds, and even tree trunks to use in your workout. A quick 30-minute outdoor workout might look something like this:

- **warm-up—5 minutes total:**

  - trail jogging

- **four main cycles—1 minute per exercise, 5 minutes per cycle:**

  - burpees

  - mountain climbers

  - high knees

  - playground pull-ups

  - park bench step-ups

- **cooldown—5 minutes total:**

    ○ walking

    ○ quad stretching

    ○ neck and shoulder stretching

    ○ chest openers

    ○ standing forward fold

Plane, Bus, and Car Workouts

By now, you know that you can work out anywhere, anytime. The tight spaces you might find yourself in—like the seat of an airplane or car—are no excuse for missing an opportunity to get your blood pumping. Note: You should not try to work out while driving yourself! If you're a passenger, on the other hand, feel free to do as many exercises as you'd like. Using some of the more discreet exercises in our list, a transit-workout may look something like this:

- **warm-up—5 minutes total:**

    ○ deep breathing

    ○ arm circles

    ○ ankle rotations

- **four main cycles—1 minute per exercise, 5 minutes per cycle:**

  - torso twists

  - shoulder blade squeezes

  - seated leg raises

  - calf raises—if you can stand up

  - standing or sitting abdominal contractions

- **cooldown—5 minutes total:**

  - seat squeezes

  - standing forward fold

  - chest opener stretch

Resistance Band Workout

So far, we've only talked about bodyweight exercises. However, even in tight spaces and during transit, you may still have a little bit of room to carry some resistance bands with you. These are basically giant rubber bands that you can use to give your workouts a little extra oomph.

When you're in your next hotel, try some of these resistance band variations in your subsequent routine:

- **Resistance band pull-aparts:** Start by holding a resistance band in front of you with both hands, arms fully extended, and hands shoulder-width apart. Stand with your feet hip-width apart, keeping a slight bend in your elbows. Engage your core for stability. While keeping your arms straight, pull the band apart by moving your hands toward the sides, squeezing your shoulder blades together. Maintain control throughout the movement and focus on using the muscles in your upper back. Resistance band pull-aparts are excellent for targeting the muscles in the upper back, specifically the rear deltoids and rhomboids. Adjust the resistance by choosing a band with an appropriate level of tension, and include this exercise in your routine to enhance shoulder stability and posture.

- **Banded squats:** To perform squats with resistance bands, begin by placing a resistance band just above your knees or around your thighs, depending on the desired level of resistance. Stand with your feet shoulder-width apart, ensuring the band is taut. You can also step on the band with both feet if you want to increase the difficulty. Engage your core, maintain an upright posture, and lower your body into a squat position by bending your knees and pushing your hips back. Keep your knees aligned with your toes and press through your heels as you return to the starting position, resisting the pull of the band. The resistance band adds extra tension throughout the movement, intensifying the workout for your glutes, hamstrings, and quadriceps.

- **Bicep curls with bands:** Start by placing the resistance band securely under both feet, ensuring it's evenly centered. Hold one end of the band in each hand, with your palms facing forward and elbows close to your sides. Stand with your feet shoulder-width apart, maintaining a slight bend in your knees for stability. Begin the curl by flexing your elbows, bringing your hands toward your shoulders while keeping your upper arms stationary. Squeeze your biceps at the top of the movement and then lower your hands back down, extending your elbows. Control the band's resistance throughout the exercise.

- **Banded tricep extensions:** Banded tricep extensions are a fantastic exercise to target and strengthen the triceps, and they can be easily done with the assistance of a resistance band. Begin by securing the band around a sturdy anchor or object above head height. Hold the other ends of the band with each hand so your arms are bent more than 90°. Slightly lean forward, with palms facing down. Slowly push down on your palms by flexing your triceps. Keep pushing down until your elbows almost lock. Return to the starting point in a controlled movement. Repeat this for however many repetitions you'd like, adjusting the tension of the band to match your strength level.

- **Single-arm row with a band:** Single-arm rows with bands target the muscles in your upper back, particularly the lats. Begin by securing a resistance band around a sturdy anchor or post at about waist height. Stand facing the anchor, holding the band in one hand with your arm fully extended. Take a step back to create tension in the band, keeping your feet shoulder-width apart. Hinge at your hips, maintain a flat back, and slightly bend your knees. Pull the band toward your hip by retracting your shoulder blade and bending your elbow, keeping it close to your body. Pause at the top of the movement, then slowly extend your arm to return to the starting position. Adjust the band's resistance to match your strength level.

Conclusion

Throughout the past 10 chapters, we've touched on a variety of subjects. From workout structures to scheduling, from creating workouts to working out on the road, one thing is certain: You now have access to a wide array of tools, both mentally and physically. When challenges arise and you start to lose motivation, simply look in your metaphorical toolbox.

The very first of your tools should be this: Fitness is possible anywhere, anytime, regardless of other factors. As such, shorter workouts and gym-free workouts are some of the best options for busy professionals, especially those who don't have time or energy to spare. Essentially, we've explored an alternative definition of fitness, one that doesn't rely on strict routines or staff scheduling. In today's working landscape, with more metrics and a bigger push for productivity every day, this is crucial. More than anything else, it's important to remember that fitness isn't just a checked box, nor is it an activity with location restraints. As long as you're willing and able, exercise is something you can do anywhere, anytime, even for the busiest of businesspeople. In essence, fitness is not merely a luxury for those who can afford it but an essential investment in your overall success and well-being. By incorporating regular exercise into your routines, you can cultivate the physical and mental resilience needed to thrive in your career, navigate challenges effectively, and achieve a sustainable work-life balance.

Now, there's only one question left to answer: Are you ready to embrace your new fitness lifestyle?

About the Author

Mark Pasay founded Rip Toned Fitness in 2013. His company creates gym gear, supplements, audio, video, and written content that helps people worldwide achieve their fitness goals. Mark is a lifelong fitness enthusiast who loves sports, travel, and concerts. He is a proud father of four and lives in BC, Canada.

Mark has been actively pursuing his own personal fitness for over 40 years now and encourages you to join him on his journey.

Learn more about Mark Pasay at https://riptoned.com

Time Crunch Fitness

Bonus Content

As an added bonus I have put together a special webpage filled with bonus content and materials to help you in your fitness journey:

Demonstration quick-workout exercise videos

Workout program videos

PDF guides for various fitness topics

Advanced exercises for when you're ready for the next level

Advanced exercise programs for when you need an extra challenge

More exercises and programs are being added regularly

Visit https://lift.riptoned.com/crunch or scan the QR code below for free access.

References

American Heart Association Recommendations for Physical Activity in Adults and Kids. (2018, April 18). American Heart Association. https://www.heart.org/en/healthy-living/fitness/fitness-basics/aha-recs-for-physical-activity-in-adults

Braun, A. (2022, July 18). *Aerobic Capacity: Definition, Ways to Improve, and More*. Verywell Health. https://www.verywellhealth.com/aerobic-capacity-5509486

Chunn, L. (2017, May 10). *The psychology of the to-do list – why your brain loves ordered tasks*. The Guardian. https://www.theguardian.com/lifeandstyle/2017/may/10/the-psychology-of-the-to-do-list-why-your-brain-loves-ordered-tasks

Clark, J. (2016). The impact of duration on effectiveness of exercise, the implication for periodization of training and goal setting for individuals who are overfat, a meta-analysis. *Biology of Sport*, *33*(4), 309–333. https://doi.org/10.5604/20831862.1212974

Cook, B. (2021, December 3). *10 ways to track fitness progress*. Stamina Products. https://staminaproducts.com/blog/10-ways-to-track-fitness-progress/

Cronkleton, E. (2022, April 29). *6 Ways to Bust Through a Workout Plateau*. Healthline.

https://www.healthline.com/nutrition/workout-plateau#how-to-break-it

Curley, B. (2020, December 18). *Gym Rat No More: 18 At-Home Exercises to Build Muscle*. Greatist. https://greatist.com/fitness/exercises-at-home-to-build-muscle#build-muscle-without-weights

de Araujo, G. G., Papoti, M., dos Reis, I. G. M., de Mello, M. A. R., & Gobatto, C. A. (2016). Short and Long Term Effects of High-Intensity Interval Training on Hormones, Metabolites, Antioxidant System, Glycogen Concentration, and Aerobic Performance Adaptations in Rats. *Frontiers in Physiology, 7.* https://doi.org/10.3389/fphys.2016.00505

English, A. (2023, January 18). *How long it takes to start seeing workout results, according to personal trainers*. Business Insider. https://www.businessinsider.com/guides/health/fitness/workout-results

Exercise and mental health. (2021, December 20). Better Health Channel. https://www.betterhealth.vic.gov.au/health/healthyliving/exercise-and-mental-health

Fatigue. (2012). Better Health Channel. https://www.betterhealth.vic.gov.au/health/conditionsandtreatments/fatigue

The 5 Basic Principles of Nutrition. (2021, September 6). Humaritarian Global.

https://humanitarianglobal.com/the-5-basic-principles-
of-nutrition/

Glycogen: What It Is & Function. (2022, July 13). Cleveland Clinic.
https://my.clevelandclinic.org/health/articles/23509-
glycogen

Golen, T., & Ricciotti, H. (2021, July 1). *Does exercise really boost
energy levels?* Harvard Health.
https://www.health.harvard.edu/exercise-and-
fitness/does-exercise-really-boost-energy-levels

Goolsby, M. A. (2021, August 16). *Overtraining: What It Is,
Symptoms, and Recovery.* Hospital for Special Surgery.
https://www.hss.edu/article_overtraining.asp

Gough, C. (2023, October 16). *US fitness industry enterprises 2022.*
Statista.
https://www.statista.com/statistics/605240/us-fitness-
health-club-industry-enterprises/

Industry Market Research, Reports, and Statistics. (2023, November
27). IBISWorld. https://www.ibisworld.com/industry-
statistics/number-of-businesses/gym-health-fitness-
clubs-united-
states/#:~:text=There%20are%20113%2C326%20Gy
m%2C%20Health

Jones, H. (2020, June 27). *10 Best Calendar Apps for Fitness
Fanatics.* Calendar. https://www.calendar.com/blog/10-
best-calendar-apps-for-fitness-fanatics/

Kamb, S. (2019, January 21). *How to Build Your Own Workout
Routine.* Nerd Fitness.

https://www.nerdfitness.com/blog/how-to-build-your-own-workout-routine

Kamb, S. (2023, October 17). *The 8 Best at Home Workouts (No-Equipment!).* NerdFitness. https://www.nerdfitness.com/blog/the-7-best-at-home-workout-routines-the-ultimate-guide-for-training-without-a-gym/#bonus_workout

Khoo, I. (2020, February 27). *How These People With Demanding Jobs Find Time For Exercise.* HuffPost. https://www.huffpost.com/archive/ca/entry/busy-schedule-workout-plan_ca_5e57dc90c5b66137fb5f1e95

Langer Research Associates. (2020). *Americans Feel Sleepy 3 Days a Week, With Impacts on Activities, Mood & Acuity.* National Sleep Foundation. https://www.thensf.org/wp-content/uploads/2020/03/SIA-2020-Report.pdf

McDonald's Restaurant Development. (2016). McDonald's. https://www.mcdonalds.com/content/dam/sites/usa/nfl/documents/franchising/mcd-site-criteria-brochure.pdf

Mirgain, S. (2018, October 11). *Resetting Your Fitness Mindset.* uwhealth. https://www.uwhealth.org/news/resetting-your-fitness-mindset

Moore, P. (2023, May 31). *Time Crunched? Your Workout Doesn't Need To Be an Hour Long, Say Experts.* The Output. https://www.onepeloton.com/blog/how-long-should-a-workout-be/

Ng, K. (2023, September 4). *This Is How many times a week you need to workout to get fit*. The Independent. https://www.independent.co.uk/life-style/health-and-families/7-minute-workout-weekly-routine-weight-loss-b2404386.html

Number of Burger King locations in the USA in 2024. (2024, January 10). ScrapeHero. https://www.scrapehero.com/location-reports/Burger%20King-USA/#:~:text=There%20are%206%2C729%20Burger%20King

Number of Pizza Hut locations in the USA in 2023. (2024, January 23). ScrapeHero. https://www.scrapehero.com/location-reports/Pizza%20Hut-USA/#:~:text=How%20many%20Pizza%20Hut%20restaurants

Number of Starbucks locations in the USA in 2024. (2024, January 29). ScrapeHero. https://www.scrapehero.com/location-reports/Starbucks-USA/#:~:text=There%20are%2016%2C386%20Starbucks%20stores

Office of Dietary Supplements - Dietary Supplements: What You Need to Know. (2020, September 3). National Institutes of Health. https://ods.od.nih.gov/factsheets/WYNTK-Consumer/

105 Hospital Statistics & Facts: How Many Hospitals Are There? (2023, November 30). Golden Steps ABA.

https://www.goldenstepsaba.com/resources/hospital-statistics-facts#:~:text=As%20of%202021%2C%20there%20are

Patton, J. (2022, May 18). *Strength Times Two*. Experience Life. https://experiencelife.lifetime.life/article/strength-times-two/

Poon, L. (2019, January 16). *Are you a robot?* Bloomberg. https://www.bloomberg.com/news/articles/2019-01-16/here-s-how-quickly-people-ditch-weight-loss-resolutions

Selhub, E. (2015, November 16). *Nutritional psychiatry: Your brain on food*. Harvard Health Blog. https://www.health.harvard.edu/blog/nutritional-psychiatry-your-brain-on-food-201511168626#:~:text=Multiple%20studies%20have%20found%20a

Setting up the Perfect Home Workout Space. You Move Me. https://youmoveme.com/blog/setting-up-the-perfect-home-workout-space/

Sleep hygiene tips - sleep and sleep disorders. (2022, September 13). Centers for Disease Control and Prevention. https://www.cdc.gov/sleep/about_sleep/sleep_hygiene.html

Statista Research Department. (2023, November 13). *Number of Subway restaurants US 2021*. Statista. https://www.statista.com/statistics/469341/number-of-subway-restaurants-

us/#:~:text=Global%20quick%20service%20restauran
t%20(QSR

Suni, E. (2020, August 14). *What is Sleep Hygiene?* (N. Vyas, Ed.).
Sleep   Foundation.
https://www.sleepfoundation.org/sleep-hygiene

*Target Heart Rate and Estimated Maximum Heart Rate | Physical
Activity.*   (2020,   September   17).   CDC.
https://www.cdc.gov/physicalactivity/basics/measurin
g/heartrate.htm#:~:text=You%20can%20estimate%20
your%20maximum

Tello, M. (2017, October 30). *Fitting in fitness for busy people.*
Harvard   Health   Blog.
https://www.health.harvard.edu/blog/fitting-in-
fitness-for-busy-people-2017103012633

U.S. and World Population Clock. (2023). United States Census
Bureau. https://www.census.gov/popclock/

Young, J. R. (n.d.). *Forbes Marketplace: 8 Time Management
Techniques For Busy People.* Forbes. Retrieved January 26,
2024,   from
https://www.forbes.com/sites/forbesmarketplace/202
1/01/20/8-time-management-techniques-for-busy-
people/?sh=258f1c7461e5